A USMLE STEP 1 REVIEW

Physiology
9th Edition

700
Questions & Answers

David G. Penney, BS, MS, PhD
*Professor of Physiology and
Occupational and Environmental Health
Wayne State University School of Medicine
Detroit, Michigan*

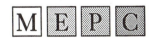

MEPC

APPLETON & LANGE
Stamford, Connecticut

Notice: The author and the publisher of this volume have taken care to make certain that the doses of drugs and schedules of treatment are correct and compatible with the standards generally accepted at the time of publication. Nevertheless, as new information becomes available, changes in treatment and in the use of drugs become necessary. The reader is advised to carefully consult the instruction and information material included in the package insert of each drug or therapeutic agent before administration. This advice is especially important when using new or infrequently used drugs. The publisher disclaims any liability, loss, injury, or damage incurred as a consequence, directly or indirectly, or the use and application of any of the contents of the volume.

Prentice Hall International (UK) Limited, *London*
Prentice Hall of Australia Pty. Limited, *Sydney*
Prentice Hall Canada. Inc., *Toronto*
Prentice Hall Hispanoamericana. S.A., *Mexico*
Prentice Hall of India Private Limited, *New Delhi*
Prentice Hall of Japan, Inc., *Tokyo*
Simon & Schuster Asia Pte. Ltd., *Singapore*
Editora Prentice Hall do Brasil Ltda., *Rio de Janeiro*
Prentice Hall, *Englewood Cliffs, New Jersey*

ISBN 0-8385-6222-1

90000

9 780838 562222

ISBN: 0-8385-6222-1

Acquisitions Editor: Marinita Timban
Production Service: Inkwell Publishing Services
Designer: Mary Skudlarek

PRINTED IN THE UNITED STATES OF AMERICA

Contents

Preface

The review of well-crafted examination questions can be a valuable learning tool in any discipline of study. This ninth edition of *Physiology* has been designed to do just that for medical students. To this end, *Physiology* has been completely revised and updated to provide questions in the current formats used on the United States Medical Licensing Examination (USMLE), Step 1.

The range of item subjects was chosen to complement and blanket the content outline of the National Board of Medical Examiners. This roster, in turn, reflects the wide scope and depth of basic science subjects taught in most medical schools today.

The question items presented are of two types: multiple choice, usually containing five distractors, and extended matching, containing as many as 20 distractors. The latter is a new format introduced to the USMLE during the past four years. Practice in working with extended matching questions will prepare the student for this format on the exam. As additional study aids, a commentary and several references follow each question, providing insight into why each distractor is either correct or incorrect, as well as giving textbook sources for further in-depth study.

By using this book, you will readily identify areas of strength and weakness in your command of various physiology subjects. Taken together, the questions and answers emphasize problem solving and the application and integration of underlying principles, as well as the retention of essential factual knowledge.

David G. Penney, PhD, Professor
Wayne State University School of Medicine
June 1995

1

Overview of Physiology

MULTIPLE CHOICE

DIRECTIONS (Questions 1–58): Each of the questions or incomplete statements below is followed by five suggested answers or completions. Select the **one** that is **best** in each case.

1. Which of the following can be said with regard to the esophagus?
   A. Conduction of food through the esophagus is controlled by vagal reflexes
   B. The upper third of the esophagus contains only smooth muscle
   C. The esophagus contains both smooth muscle and skeletal muscle
   D. Conduction of food through the esophagus is controlled primarily by enteric reflexes originating in the esophagus
   E. C and D are correct

2. Which of the following may increase the force-generating capacity of a muscle?
   A. Increasing the diameter of a muscle fiber without an increase in fiber length
   B. Increasing the length of a muscle fiber without an increase in diameter
   C. Increasing connective tissue content
   D. Parallel rather than pennate arrangement of cells
   E. All are correct

3. All of the following are characteristics of muscle tissue **EXCEPT**
   A. classified anatomically and functionally
   B. chemomechanical transduction
   C. individual cells of voluntary muscle tissue are arranged in parallel and function independently
   D. individual cells of involuntary muscle tissue are arranged in parallel and cannot function independently
   E. all are correct

4. Local spinal circuitry may be influenced by axons descending from the brain. The specific effect of this influence depends on
   A. discharge properties of the descending axon
   B. location or distribution of terminal axons
   C. physiologic inhibitory effect of the axon
   D. physiologic excitatory effect of the axon
   E. all are correct

5. Body fluid pH depends primarily on the renal control of
   A. reabsorption of sodium dibasic phosphate and secretion of bicarbonate
   B. reabsorption of sodium in exchange for potassium
   C. secretion of hydrogen ion in exchange for potassium
   D. secretion of hydrogen ion in exchange for sodium
   E. secretion of hydrogen ion in exchange for calcium

6. The function(s) of the gallbladder include
   A. equalization of pressure in bile duct system
   B. reduction of alkalinity of bile pH
   C. concentration of bile fluid
   D. A and B are correct
   E. all are correct

7. The effects of spinal transection include all of the following **EXCEPT**
    A. permanent anesthesia to body parts innervated by segments below transection
    B. permanent loss of somatic reflexes below transection
    C. permanent paralysis of voluntary musculature innervated by segments below transection
    D. permanent loss of autonomic reflexes below transection
    E. A and C are correct

8. The lens of the eye
    A. has a shorter focal length when relaxed
    B. has a fatter conformity when relaxed
    C. experiences less tension from support fibers when relaxed
    D. is not relaxed during accommodation
    E. B and D are correct

9. Neuropeptides are found throughout the nervous system and play a central role in synaptic transmission. Some neuropeptides serve as neuromodulators whose functions include
    A. amplification of postsynaptic response
    B. reduction of postsynaptic response
    C. A and B are correct
    D. increase-voltage of postsynaptic response
    E. all are correct

10. The primary cause(s) of heat stroke is(are)
    A. excessive heat production
    B. inability to sweat
    C. conductive heat gain
    D. inability to lose heat by radiation
    E. convective heat gain

11. Which of the following is (are) true regarding the chemical sensory mechanisms?
    A. Limited to sensory mechanisms associated with taste
    B. Include chemoreceptors located on the tongue and in the larynx and pharnyx
    C. Limited to the olfactory sensory mechanisms
    D. Limited to the sense of smell
    E. None are correct

12. Properties of mediated transport include
    A. saturation kinetics exhibited
    B. transport across membrane at rates faster than predicted for molecules of similar size and lipid solubility
    C. exhibit competitive inhibition
    D. equilibration of substrate across cell membrane as in facilitated transport
    E. all are correct

13. In general, in receptive fields
    A. transducer-containing tissue maintains its electrochemical properties in response to a stimulus
    B. a particular transducing tissue is relatively insensitive in that it is nonspecific for stimulus
    C. the transducer tissue response will perceive a specific stimulus from extreme forms of inappropriate stimuli as if the appropriate stimulus were there
    D. the ability to determine how much stimuli is present is due to the adaptation phenomenon
    E. all are correct

14. The sympathetic nervous system
    A. is predominantly excitatory
    B. is involved more frequently in generalized rather than discrete discharge
    C. is of great importance in visual accommodation of the lens
    D. may antagonize parasympathetic functions
    E. A, B, and D are correct

15. Acclimatization to high altitude involves
    A. maintaining ventilation that is excessive with respect to CO_2 exchange
    B. producing an acid urine
    C. increasing the oxygen-carrying capacity of arterial blood
    D. A and C are correct
    E. all are correct

16. Which of the following is (are) generally employed for long-term reduction of acid and pepsin secretion in a duodenal ulcer patient?
    A. Complete gastrectomy
    B. Daily administration of atropine in doses sufficient to block all action of acetylcholine

C. Giving the patient plenty of aspirin in order to kill the pain, thereby reducing a stressful situation

D. Gastric vagotomy plus pyloric antrectomy

E. All are correct

17. The pyramidal tract arises from the following **EXCEPT**
    A. primary motor cortex
    B. somatic sensory areas of the cortex
    C. premotor cortex
    D. medulla
    E. none of the above

18. Stimulation of the myenteric plexus results in which of the following?
    A. Decreased velocity of conduction along the gut wall
    B. Increased "tone" of the gut wall
    C. Decreased rhythmic contractions
    D. Increased rate of rhythmic contractions of the gut wall
    E. B and D are correct

19. Properties of smooth muscle include
    A. rapid contraction with the inability of sustained tonic contraction
    B. inability for rhythmic spontaneous contraction
    C. reciprocal innervation by sympathetic and parasympathetic systems
    D. insensitivity to mechanical, thermal, and chemical stimuli
    E. A and C are correct

20. With regard to gastric emptying
    A. the driving force of the emptying process is the pressure differential between the gastric and duodenal side of the pylorus
    B. it is influenced by duodenal pH
    C. it requires about 1 to 3 hours for a normal fixed meal
    D. it is facilitated by parasympathetic stimulation
    E. all are correct

21. The normal fluidity of circulating blood is probably maintained by
    A. plasmin
    B. plasma antithromboplastin
    C. plasma antithrombin
    D. heparin
    E. all are correct

22. The volume of blood per total body weight
    A. is constant for all members of a species (e.g., man)
    B. varies from about 5 to 10 mL/kg
    C. is generally higher for women than for men
    D. is greater in individuals with a greater total body weight
    E. B and D are correct

23. The oxygen-carrying capacity of whole blood is
    A. about 2 vol%
    B. largely determined by the plasma protein concentration
    C. directly proportional to the hemoglobin content
    D. increased in the presence of carbon dioxide
    E. A and C are correct

24. Receptors in joints are primarily associated with
    A. somatosensation
    B. thermosensation
    C. chemosensation
    D. proprioception
    E. A and D are correct

25. Physiologic levels of both growth hormone and thyroxine
    A. decrease the rate of protein synthesis
    B. store fat in adipose tissue
    C. are necessary for normal growth and development
    D. increase the peripheral uptake and utilization of glucose
    E. A, B, and C are correct

26. Chief cells secrete
    A. zymogen granules
    B. intrinsic factor
    C. pepsinogen
    D. HCl
    E. A and C are correct

27. The collecting ducts are the site of final adjustment of urinary
    A. sodium
    B. potassium
    C. water
    D. pH
    E. all are correct

28. When using para-aminohippurate (PAH) to determine renal plasma flow (RPF) it is necessary to know which of the following values?
   A. Venous concentration of PAH
   B. Urine concentration of K^+
   C. Urinary flow rate
   D. Urine pH
   E. A and D are correct

29. The initial step in the formation of urine is considered to be ultrafiltration at the glomeruli. The forces **AIDING** ultrafiltration include
   A. colloid osmotic pressure of plasma protein
   B. glomerular capillary pressure
   C. hydrostatic pressure in Bowman's capsule
   D. crystalloid osmotic pressure of the final urine
   E. B and C are correct

30. During exercise, increased O_2 to the active muscles depends on the following factors
   A. skin temperature
   B. ventilation rate
   C. blood lactate concentration
   D. arteriovenous oxygen content difference
   E. B and D are correct

31. The carotid sinus baroreceptors in the adult human
   A. respond to relative hypoxia of the peripheral blood
   B. give rise to a depressor reflex if the blood pressure is too high
   C. are connected with cortical centers via the vagi
   D. exert discontinuous control in the vasomotor and cardioregulatory centers
   E. response to falling pressure in the same way they respond to rising pressure

32. Proteins produced by the platelets include
   A. plasminogen
   B. fibrinogen
   C. prothrombin
   D. thromboplastin
   E. albumin

33. Loss of heat occurs from the body core to the periphery and to the air by
   A. circulatory-assisted conductive and convective heat transport
   B. thermal radiation between body cells to the air
   C. the sweat glands
   D. convection from body cell to body cell and to the air
   E. A and C are correct

34. Initially, in the febrile or fever state
   A. the body loses its thermoregulatory capabilities
   B. body temperature continues to rise
   C. neurocontrol of peripheral vasculature is lost
   D. the hypothalamic set point temperature has been reset at a supernormal level
   E. A, B, and C are correct

35. The contractile muscle of the heart is like skeletal muscle in that
   A. it is cross-striated
   B. the contractile elements are formed from myosin
   C. the force of contraction is increased by stretching (within physiologic limits)
   D. it is made up of myotubes
   E. A, B, and C are correct

36. The stretch reflex will be evoked when certain receptors are affected. These are
   A. annulospiral endings
   B. flower spray endings
   C. Golgi organ
   D. Meissner's corpuscles
   E. A, B, and C are correct

37. Cellular membranes
   A. act as semipermeable barriers essential to maintaining an intracellular composition different from the outside environment
   B. are responsible for forming compartments within cells
   C. A and B are correct
   D. vary in function, but structure and composition are the same among membranes of a single cell and from cell to cell
   E. all are correct

38. Prolonged hyperventilation may lead to respiratory alkalosis. This condition may be associated with
   A. increased renal reabsorption of bicarbonate
   B. decreased renal excretion of ammonium ion
   C. dissociation of acid buffers
   D. raising of plasma bicarbonate concentration
   E. B and D are correct

39. A pure tone can be characterized by
   A. frequency and amplitude only
   B. amplitude and phase only
   C. phase only
   D. frequency, amplitude, and phase
   E. none of the above

40. Opioids
   A. are called morphine-like because they produce responses similar to morphine
   B. are produced in the central nervous system
   C. are produced in the pituitary gland
   D. seem to illicit complex behavioral changes including changes in mood and response to pain and stress
   E. all are correct

41. Which is not a function of the vestibular system?
   A. Senses forces in linear and rotational acceleration
   B. Stabilizes eye position
   C. Spatial displacement of sound
   D. A and B are correct
   E. A and C are correct

42. During excess intake of fluids the extra volume of water is located predominantly in the
   A. intravascular compartment
   B. intracellular compartment
   C. interstitial compartment
   D. transvascular (GI tract and cerebrospinal fluid) compartment
   E. A and C are correct

43. Which of the following is a function of the cerebellum?
  A. Coordination and modulation of muscular activity
  B. Execution of body movement
  C. Integration of information concerning body position, muscle tension, and muscle length on a moment-to-moment basis
  D. Responsible for nonproprioceptive information
  E. A and C are correct

44. Swallowing
  A. is strictly under voluntary control
  B. is strictly under involuntary control
  C. takes place in two stages: the voluntary stage and the pharyngeal stage
  D. inhibits respiration during the pharyngeal stage
  E. A and C are correct

45. To minimize sweating during exposure to the sun in a hot desert, one should
  A. wear as much black clothing as possible to reflect the rays
  B. remove clothing and walk slowly to increase convection currents
  C. walk clothed
  D. sit quietly and clothed (in white color and of texture that permits air flow)
  E. none are correct

46. Under normal external temperature conditions, the most important system controlling water excretion or loss is
  A. skin
  B. lungs
  C. kidneys
  D. gastrointestinal tract
  E. body hair

47. Salivary secretion
  A. is only affected by parasympathetic innervation
  B. contains an enzyme that must be stored in zymogen granules before it is secreted
  C. is stimulated by sympathetic innervation
  D. contains the enzyme salivary amylase
  E. is a passive process and does not involve any enzymatic processes

48. Which of the following is most related to the fact that, in the steady state, cell membranes are relatively more permeable to potassium than to sodium?

  A. Cells possess an outside-negative transmembrane resting potential

  B. Cells possess an inside-negative transmembrane resting potential

  C. Cells change volume in the presence of somatic pressure gradients

  D. Normal cells show a progressive diminution in the internal potassium concentration in the steady state

  E. Cells do not possess active ion transport systems

49. In negative water balance

  A. the cells and extracellular compartment are hydrated

  B. only the cells are hydrated

  C. the intracellular compartment is hydrated but the extracellular compartment is dehydrated

  D. the total body water content is reduced

  E. the cells and extracellular compartment are dehydrated

50. A sample of human erythrocytes is placed into a solution of plasma that has been made hyperosmotic with the addition of urea, a substance that is permeable to the red blood cell (RBC) membrane. Which of the following best describes the results?

  A. The cells would shrink transiently and tend to return their normal volume

  B. The cells would swell and hemolyze

  C. The cells would shrink and then swell and hemolyze

  D. No change in the cell volume would be observed at any time

  E. The cells would undergo rapid mitosis

51. Which of the following is **NOT** associated with orthostatic hypotension?

  A. Increased heart rate

  B. Constriction of visceral and skeletal muscle arterioles

  C. Increased sympathetic activity

  D. Increased respiratory depth

  E. Venoconstriction

52. Sebaceous glands
    A. arise independent of the follicular canal
    B. secrete sebum from a single layer of basal cells that line their lumen
    C. increase their activity under the influence of androgens
    D. secrete sebum only in response to adrenergic excitation
    E. are important for temperature control

53. The primary stimulus for increasing heat loss to maintain thermal homeostasis arises from
    A. temperature receptors in the skin
    B. cold receptors in the skin
    C. special thermal receptors in the veins
    D. special thermal receptors in the arteries
    E. the anterior hypothalamus following elevated temperatures above a specific value

54. Which of the following best describes the process of diffusion?
    A. A "downhill" process that is passive in nature (no metabolic energy is necessary)
    B. An "uphill" process that is active in nature requiring a metabolic energy input
    C. A driven process that is purely dependent upon the presence of a true driving force such as a pressure or voltage gradient
    D. A process by which only large molecular weight proteins may move across biologic membranes
    E. Requires metabolic energy

55. In Figure 1 assume that side A is the capillary, side B the interstitial fluid, and the line separating compartments A and B the vessel wall. In such a situation, which of the following statements is **INCORRECT**?
    A. The protein in the capillaries is relatively impermeable and will stay in the vessel
    B. The H_2O in side B will tend to diffuse into side A due to the plasma oncotic colloid osmotic pressure
    C. Any pathologic situation that causes the vascular protein to enter side B would result in the clinical condition of edema

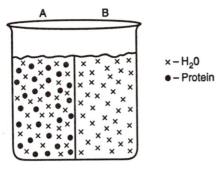

Figure 1

D. The capillary hydrostatic pressure would oppose H_2O filtration from side B to side A

E. None of the above are correct because in all living organisms the capillary proteins are freely diffusible and hence would come to osmotic equilibrium

56. The best evidence that the plasma clearance of inulin (C_{in}) measures glomerular filtration rate in man is
   A. at high urine flows the clearance of urea approaches C_{in}
   B. it is found in the urine of aglomerular kidneys
   C. when phlorizin is given glucose and creatinine have the same clearance as inulin
   D. when the tubules are overloaded with para-aminohippurate (PAH) the clearance of PAH approaches C_{in}
   E. at low urine flows the clearance of glucose approaches C_{in}

57. Heparin prevents clotting primarily because it
   A. dissolves fibrinogen
   B. blocks conversion of prothrombin to thrombin
   C. inactivates thromboplastin
   D. chelates calcium
   E. blocks the action of thrombin

58. In a patient with diabetes mellitus who has a high blood glucose level and a filtered load of glucose above tubular transport maximum (T_m) level
   A. the polydipsia leads to plasma dilution, decreased plasma osmolality, and hyponatremia
   B. retention of sodium in exchange for potassium leads to a hypokalemic, metabolic acidosis
   C. the osmotic diuresis leads to a hyponatremic dehydration due to loss of sodium in excess of water
   D. there is base (sodium) conservation with reabsorption of bicarbonate in preference to chloride and resultant metabolic alkalosis
   E. there is metabolic acidosis that may be complicated by potassium retention since hydrogen is selectively secreted by the distal nephron in exchange for sodium

MATCHING

DIRECTIONS (Questions 59–77): Each group of questions below consists of a set of lettered components, followed by a list of numbered words or phrases. For **each** numbered word or phrase, select the **one** lettered component that is most closely associated with it. Each lettered component may be selected once, more than once, or not at all.

Questions 59–63 (Figure 2):

   A. phase 4
   B. phase 2
   C. phase 3
   D. phase 0
   E. phase 1

In Figure 2,

59. deflection #6 is

60. deflection #7 is

61. deflection #8 is

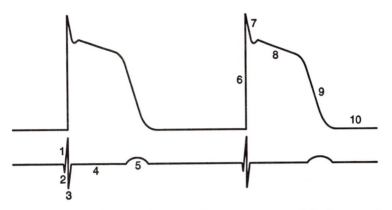

Figure 2 Recordings of the intracellular action potentials (top trace) and simultaneous electrographic tracings (bottom trace) from ventricular contractile tissue.

62. deflection #9 is

63. deflection #10 is

Questions 64–70 (Figure 3):

    A. K^+ efflux
    B. Cl^- influx
    C. fast Na^+ influx
    D. slow Ca^{2+} influx
    E. slow Ca^{2+} influx and simultaneous K^+ efflux

In Figure 3, the ionic movement responsible for current #1 is

64. current #1 is

65. current #2 is

66. current #4 is

67. current #5 is

68. current #7 is

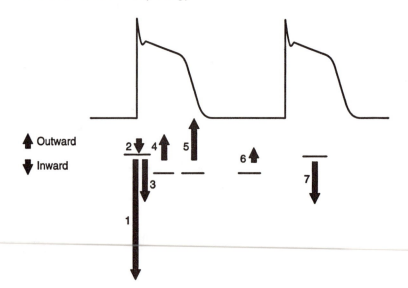

Figure 3 Arrows indicate the direction of current flow carried by ionic movement.

69. current #3 is

70. current #6 is

Questions 71 and 72 (Figure 4):

    A. curve A
    B. curve B

In Figure 4, the curve which represents the relationship between pressure and flow for

71. an atherosclerotic (rigid) artery is

72. a normal distensible artery is

Questions 73–77 (Figure 5):

    A. site A
    B. site B
    C. site C
    D. site D

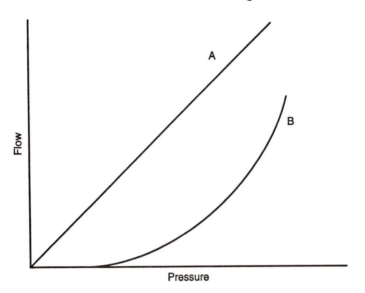

Figure 4 Pressure-flow relationship of the blood in two different vessels.

In Figure 5, the site(s) at which there occurs the greatest or highest

73. urea concentration is

74. K^+ reabsorption is

75. K^+ secretion is

76. creatinine secretion is

77. activity of antidiuretic hormone (ADH) is

Figure 5 Schematic representation of a normal renal tubule.

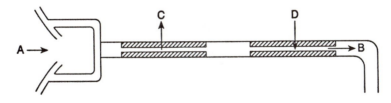

DIRECTIONS (Questions 78–87): Each group of questions below consists of a diagram with lettered components, followed by a list of numbered words or phrases. For **each** numbered word or phrase, select the **one** lettered component that is most closely associated with it. Each lettered component may be selected once, more than once, or not at all.

Questions 78–80 (Figure 6):

78. action potential (voltage alterations)

79. conductance changes exhibited by sodium (Na$^+$)

80. conductance changes exhibited by potassium (K$^+$)

Questions 81–87 (Figure 7):

81. local response

82. negative afterpotential

83. overshoot

Figure 6 Relationship between membrane conductance and membrane voltage alterations as a function of time following a depolarization.

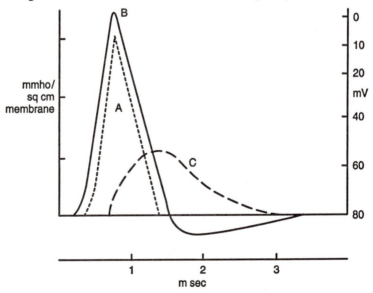

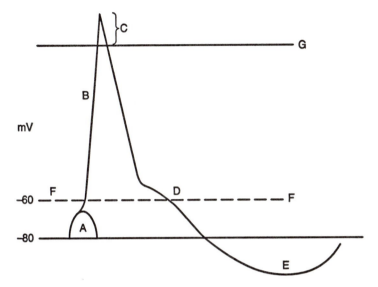

Figure 7 Representation of a nerve action potential.

84. spike potential

85. positive afterpotential

86. level of potential at which the depolarizing process becomes self-generative (threshold potential)

87. level at which no voltage gradient is present across the membrane

Overview of Physiology

Answers and Discussion

1. **(E)** The esophagus is a muscular tube that conducts fluids and solids from the pharynx to the stomach during the third stage of swallowing. In humans, the upper third is skeletal muscle and during resting conditions is closed owing to the tonic contractions of the pharyngoesophageal sphincter. This prevents air from entering the esophagus during inspiration. Near the stomach region the esophageal muscles are of the smooth type and are not under conscious control. Initiation of the swallowing reflex is controlled by the vagus and the peristaltic conduction of food through the esophagus is primarily a continuation of contractions initiated in the pharynx. However, if primary peristalsis fails to move food through the esophagus, enteric reflexes originating in the esophagus take over. (**Ref. 2,** pp. 448–450)

2. **(A)** Increasing the diameter (hypertrophy) will increase the force generated by the muscle regardless of length. However, increasing the length by addition of sarcomeres without a change in diameter leaves the force-generating capacity unchanged. Most cells are arranged at an angle to the axes of the muscle, an arrangement which allows more fibers to attach to the tendon and increases total force-generating capacity. (**Ref. 1,** pp. 300–301)

3. **(E)** Muscle is responsible for chemomechanical transduction; conversion of chemical energy into mechanical energy. Muscle tissue is classified primarily two different ways: according to anato-

my (smooth versus striated) and according to function (voluntary versus involuntary). Involuntary muscle cells are arranged in series as well as in parallel, forming a sheet of muscle. Consequently, the cells cannot function independently. (**Ref. 1,** pp. 281–291)

4. **(E)** The physiologic effect of descending axons on local spinal circuitry may be inhibitory or excitatory. This is influenced, of course, by location or distribution of axons and their discharge properties. (**Ref. 2,** pp. 184–191)

5. **(D)** The entire nephron is geared primarily for active transport involving Na^+, H^+ exchange. Substitutes for Na^+ by other ions do occur, but these are secondary. Although H^+ secretion is determined by plasma K, it is the kidney which controls pH. (**Ref. 2,** pp. 641–665)

6. **(E)** The major function is one of bile concentration. Other subsidiary functions include an ability to reduce bile alkalinity and the equalization of pressure within the bile system. The pressure equalization would be minimal or negligible if the gallbladder could not reabsorb fluid and reduce the bulk of the bile. (**Ref. 2,** pp. 458–463)

7. **(E)** Spinal transection results in immediate paralysis of all muscles innervated by spinal segments below the transection site. There is anesthesia in all body parts accordingly. However, although the somatic reflexes, such as muscle tone and the withdrawal response, along with the autonomic responses, may be abolished as well by transection, the loss is transient and is usually recovered, depending on the level of transection. (**Ref. 2,** pp. 184–194)

8. **(D)** Relaxation principally refers to the circular musculature (ciliary body) around the lens to which tough support fibers (zonular fibers) are attached. In the relaxed state, tension from these fibers pulls the lens flat. Contraction of the ciliary bodies during accommodation relieves tension of the zonular fibers and the lens assumes a more spherical shape, which allows for closer focusing. (**Ref. 2,** pp. 137–140)

9. **(C)** Though neuromodulators may prolong, shorten, reduce, and amplify the postsynaptic response, they do not cause substantive change in conduction or voltage. (**Ref. 2**, pp. 96–99)

10. **(B)** Heat stroke is caused by failure of the sweating mechanisms. The reasons for this malfunction are not well understood. (**Ref. 2**, pp. 227–232)

11. **(B)** Olfaction (smell) and gustation (taste) are the only senses that can identify chemical stimuli. Chemoreceptors for taste can be found throughout the mouth, including the larynx and pharnyx. Of all the senses, olfaction is the least understood for at least two reasons. There are no odors analogous to sweet, sour, bitter, or salty taste. Second, sensory pathways themselves are difficult to characterize because of their diffuse nature. (**Ref. 2**, pp. 167–170)

12. **(E)** All these properties are distinguishing features of mediated transport and are common to both active and facilitated transport. The distinguishing feature between these two is simply that active transport will "pump" against a concentration gradient whereas facilitated transport tends to equilibrate substances across the membrane. (**Ref. 2**, pp. 22–27)

13. **(C)** Transducer-containing tissue generally responds to a stimulus through electrochemical means. This response is relatively sensitive to one specific form of stimulus. Therefore, an inappropriate stimulus, if strong enough, will be perceived as the appropriate response. For example, if enough pressure is applied to the eye the retina will perceive the stimulus as flashes of light and not a mechanical stimulus. These tissues have developed not only the ability to determine how much stimuli is present but, through spatial distribution, can determine where the stimuli is located. However, slow adaptation sacrifices some precision in the intensity code in favor of an increased dynamic range. (**Ref. 2**, pp. 105–110)

14. **(E)** The excitatory sympathetic nervous system is involved more frequently in generalized rather than discrete discharge. It is of little importance in visual accommodation of the lens and antagonizes some parasympathetic functions. (**Ref. 2**, pp. 203–205)

15. **(D)** Acclimatization to high altitude involves maintaining ventilation that is excessive with respect to CO_2 exchanges and increasing the oxygen capacity of arterial blood. An alkaline urine is produced. (**Ref. 2,** pp. 627–630)

16. **(D)** The performance of a vagotomy will lessen the secretion of acid and pepsin by the stomach. The pyloric antrectomy is necessary to compensate for the decrease in the rate of gastric emptying. (**Ref. 2,** pp. 450–456)

17. **(D)** Sixty percent of the pyramidal tract (also called the corticospinal tract) originates from the primary motor cortex, with 20% from the premotor cortex and 20% from the somatic sensory areas of the cortex. After leaving the cortex, the pyramidal tract passes through the brain stem, forming the pyramids of the medulla, then down into the corticospinal tracts. (**Ref. 2,** pp. 185–188)

18. **(E)** Stimulation of the myenteric plexus increases motor activity in the manner indicated in the question (i.e., increased tone, rhythm, rate, and velocity of contraction of the gut wall). (**Ref. 2,** pp. 442–443)

19. **(C)** Smooth muscle is capable of sustained tonic contraction, although it is slow and sluggish. It is capable of rhythmic spontaneous contraction and it is innervated reciprocally by sympathetic and parasympathetic systems. (**Ref. 2,** pp. 71–74)

20. **(E)** Gastric emptying is influenced by duodenal pH and is facilitated by parasympathetic stimulation. Emptying takes about 1 to 3 hours for a normal meal. The driving force of the emptying process is the pressure differential between the gastric and the duodenal side of the pylorus. (**Ref. 2,** pp. 450–451)

21. **(E)** All the listed elements contribute to the maintenance of fluid blood. (**Ref. 2,** pp. 473–478)

22. **(D)** The volume of blood per total body weight will vary considerably from one individual to another, but it will be roughly

proportional to body weight. Blood volume varies between 70 and 90 mL/kg. (Ref. 2, pp. 473–474)

23. (C) The capacity of blood to bind oxygen is fairly large and is proportional to the concentration of hemoglobin. It is approximately 20 vol%. (Ref. 2, pp. 486–490)

24. (D) Proprioception is the sense of joint position. (Ref. 2, pp. 105–108)

25. (C) Physiologic levels of growth hormone and thyroxine both increase the rate of protein synthesis and mobilize fat from adipose tissue, and they are necessary for normal growth and development. (Ref. 2, pp. 372–374, 290–296)

26. (E) The major secretion of the chief cells is pepsinogen in the form of zymogen granules (Ref. 2, pp. 450–451)

27. (E) The collecting ducts of the kidney are final active areas for control of many substances found in the urine and play an important role in determining the pH of the urine. (Ref. 2, pp. 650–660)

28. (C) Effective RPF = urine concentration of PAH × urine volume/arterial concentration of PAH. (Ref. 2, pp. 645–647)

29. (B) The glomerular capillary pressure aids glomerular filtration, most of the other factors oppose filtration. (Ref. 2, pp. 647–650)

30. (E) Increased ventilation and arteriovenous oxygen difference are two of the most important factors allowing increased oxygen supply to exercising muscles. (Ref. 2, pp. 625–627, 577–579)

31. (B) The carotid sinus receptors primarily are active in the control of blood pressure and are only a secondary influence on the control of blood pO_2. They respond stronger to rising pressure than to falling pressure. (Ref. 2, pp. 549–551)

32. (D) The platelets are the site for thromboplastin production, whereas prothrombin, plasminogen, prothrombin, and albumin are synthesized in the liver. (Ref. 2, pp. 485–486)

33. **(E)** Because of the volume of the human body the circulatory-assisted conductive and convective heat transport is essential for normal maintenance of body temperature. **(Ref. 2,** pp. 229–230)

34. **(D)** The initial step in development of a febrile incident is the alteration of the set point of the hypothalamic temperature control center. **(Ref. 2,** pp. 231–232)

35. **(E)** The first three are properties shared by both muscle types. Cardiac muscle cells are not formed into myotubes as are skeletal muscle cells. **(Ref. 2,** pp. 67–71)

36. **(E)** The receptors that are needed to activate the stretch reflex are located within the muscle itself and, hence, it is the muscle receptor stimulation that induces the stretch reflex. **(Ref. 2,** pp. 113–121)

37. **(C)** Cellular membranes exhibit incredible diversity of structure, function, and composition. Though various membranes have some common features, membrane composition, and structure differ not only from cell to cell but differ among membranes within a single cell. **(Ref. 2,** pp. 4–6)

38. **(A)** Respiratory alkalosis primarily is a result of excess CO_2 that is blown off by the lungs, which results in a lower plasma bicarbonate concentration and concomitant increase in its reabsorption by the kidney. **(Ref. 2,** pp. 619–620, 672–673)

39. **(D)** Another parameter is needed to characterize sine waves, the mean level of the sine wave, "d.c." This is the average of peak to trough of the sinusoidal wave. However, in sound waves the d.c. level is not crucial as the d.c. refers to the ambient air pressure. **(Ref. 2,** pp. 154–162)

40. **(E)** Many opioids have been found to be produced in widely scattered groups of cells within the body. The distribution of these cells include the cerebral cortex and spinal chord. They also are found in many synaptic terminals and axons. Their specific function, whether analgesic or otherwise, is impossible to define for each of the opioids, but they seem to play an underlying role in the formation of complex behavior. **(Ref. 2,** pp. 97–99)

41. **(D)** The principal function of the vestibular system is to sense forces due to acceleration, both linear and rotational and particularly the linear force of gravity. Actually, the vestibular system senses head acceleration. This sensory ability serves to stabilize eye position on a fixed point even though the head may be moving. It is essential for balance and posture. Even though the vestibular system is part of the inner ear, the vestibular pathways have nothing analogous to the sense of hearing. (**Ref. 2,** pp. 164–166)

42. **(B)** The bulk of the extra water load (and up to water intoxication) moves into the cells of the blood and other tissues causing cellular hydration. (**Ref. 2,** pp. 670–672)

43. **(E)** The cerebellum is involved with regulation of movement rather than its execution. It acts as a modulator of movement to smooth and coordinate movement. Of course this requires moment-to-moment input of information, all of which must be integrated and transmitted to descending motor pathways for ongoing activity. (**Ref. 2,** pp. 197–202)

44. **(D)** Swallowing occurs primarily in three stages: the oral or voluntary, the pharyngeal, and the exophageal phase. The oral phase is strictly voluntary. However, after the bolus enters the pharyngeal stage involuntary reflexes take over. These reflexes are designed to propel the bolus towards the stomach at the same time preventing food from entering the trachea by inhibiting respiration and closing the epiglottis. This particular reflex takes place during the pharyngeal phase. (**Ref. 2,** pp. 448–450)

45. **(D)** The best ways to minimize sweating are to avoid exercise, remain clothed, and attempt to reduce (if possible) direct exposure to the sun. (**Ref. 2,** pp. 227–232)

46. **(C)** The kidneys are the supreme controllers of water excretion and account for over 60% of body water loss in the form of urine. Water loss also occurs via the lungs, skin, and the GI tract. (**Ref. 2,** pp. 641–644)

47. **(D)** The only enzyme secreted by the salivary glands is salivary amylase. (**Ref. 2,** pp. 448–450)

48. (B) The greater permeability of a membrane to potassium will allow that membrane to develop a transmembrane potential that is largely a potassium diffusion potential. (**Ref. 2,** pp. 30–31)

49. (D) By definition, when total body water is reduced the body is said to be in negative water balance. (**Ref. 2,** pp. 654–656)

50. (A) When human red cells are placed in plasma made hyperosmotic with urea the red cells will lose water until enough urea has moved into the red cell to reverse such loss. At this point, the cells will begin to return to normal size. (**Ref. 2,** pp. 28–30)

51. (D) The sudden drop in arterial pressure results in vagal withdrawal and an increase in heart rate. After a few minutes, sympathetic activity and circulating catecholamines serve to increase heart rate. However, the major effect of moving to a standing position is on the veins rather than the arterioles. Baroreceptor or chemoreceptor reflex elicits the abdominal compression reflex which helps translocate blood out of the abdominal vascular reservoirs; however, this reflex action of the abdominal muscles tends to limit rather than increase depth of respiration. (**Ref. 2,** pp. 575–576)

52. (C) Testosterone stimulates both the growth and secretion of sebaceous glands. (**Ref. 2,** pp. 395–399)

53. (E) The preoptic anterior hypothalamus is the major central area responsible for the sensing of body temperatures. (**Ref. 2,** pp. 227–232)

54. (A) Diffusion is basically a passive process that can only occur down an electrochemical gradient. (**Ref. 2,** pp. 28–31)

55. (E) The distribution of fluid and ions between the vascular and interstitial compartments is controlled by the balance between hydrostatic and osmotic forces at the capillary level. The most important force is the capillary hydrostatic pressure which promotes filtration of H_2O and the water filtration is opposed by the plasma colloid osmotic pressure. Normally the vessel wall is impermeable to proteins. But a shift in membrane permeability to favor protein entry into the tissue could cause H_2O to enter the interstitial compartment and result in edema. (**Ref. 2,** pp. 536–540)

56. **(C)** The best evidence that plasma clearance of inulin (Cin) measures glomerular filtration rate in man is when phlorizin is given. Glucose and creatinine have the same clearance as inulin. Since phlorizin blocks sugar reabsorption, their clearance should then be identical with that of inulin. (**Ref. 2,** pp. 647–648)

57. **(E)** Heparin prevents clotting primarily because it inhibits the action of thrombin on fibrinogen and thereby prevents the conversion of fibrinogen to fibrin threads. It does this by increasing the efforts of antithrombin III. (**Ref. 2,** pp. 495–496)

58. **(E)** The diabetic is constantly excreting high glucose amounts in the urine. The formation of ketones and decreased hydrogen for Na exchange yields a situation in which the patient is in a metabolic acidotic condition with loss of sodium, glucose, and large amounts of water. Since any Na^+ that is reabsorbed is exchanged for hydrogen, it leads to a K^+ retention. (**Ref. 2,** pp. 324–326)

59. **(D); 60. (E); 61. (B); 62. (C); 63. (A)** Transmembrane action potentials of the heart are descriptively labeled as phase 0 for the initial rapid depolarization (spike) including the overshoot. Phase 1 represents the initial rapid repolarization with phase 2 as the slow almost steady-state repolarization (plateau). The final repolarization curve is referred to as phase 3 which returns the membrane potential to its resting level (phase 4). (**Ref. 2,** pp. 498–500, 69–70)

64. **(C); 65. (D); 66. (A); 67. (A); 68. (D); 69. (B); 70. (A)** The cardiac action potential is a result of changes in membrane permeability to Na^+, Cl^-, Ca^{2+}, and K^+ going through "fast" or "slow" channels and controlled by "gates" which open or close in response to voltage changes. During phase 0 the Na^+ conductance is high with some influx of Ca^{2+}. Phase 1 is caused by an inward Cl^- current with a slight contribution by an outward K^+ current. The plateau or phase 2 is largely a continuous slow inward flow of Ca^{2+} with some contribution of a slow Na^+ inward. Also during phase 2 there is an anomalous rectification with K^+ moving in the outward direction. During phase 3 there is mainly a K^+ outward movement (through channels referred to as X_i). The resting level (phase 4) is maintained mainly by an outward K^+ movement. (**Ref. 2,** pp. 69–70, 498–500)

71. (A); 72. (B)   The pressure-flow relationship for distensible blood vessels is not linear but curvilinear. In rigid vessels the flow is proportional to pressure in the range of 20 and 100 mm Hg mainly because the resistance to flow is constant. In a distensible vessel the resistance is changing (1/R), which is due to a passive increase in vessel radius in response to increased pressure. As higher pressures are reached, the vessels passively dilate and thereby increase flow. So in a normal blood vessel the blood flow will increase in response to both an increased pressure and a decreased resistance, accounting for the curvilinear slope. (**Ref. 2,** pp. 529–533)

73. (B)   The body normally forms about 25 and 30 g of urea each day and probably greater amounts in individuals on very high protein diets. This urea must be excreted in the urine, otherwise uremia will develop. (Normally the plasma concentration is 26 mg/100 mL, but in patients with renal insufficiency it can go up to 200 mg/100 mL). The rate of urea excretion is dependent upon glomerular filtration rate (GFR) and plasma concentration. At normal GFR about 60% of the filtered load is passed through the tubules, being higher or lower with changes in GFR. The lower collecting duct has the highest urea concentration, which is passively reabsorbed into the medullary interstitium and causes high concentration. The urea is then reabsorbed into the thin loop of Henle, so that it passes upward through these terminal renal portions several times before it is finally excreted. Despite the recirculation, none of the urea is actually reabsorbed into the blood but is eventually excreted into the urine in a very high concentration even though little water is excreted along with it, thereby the important role of urea in the execution of highly concentrated urine. (**Ref. 2,** pp. 657–660)

74. (B)   Potassium is transported through the tubules in almost identical fashion as sodium. About 65% of filtered K^+ is reabsorbed in the proximal tubules with 25% in the dilating segment of the distal tubules. By the end of the distal tubule only 10% of filtered K^+ is left. (**Ref. 2,** pp. 650–654)

75. (D)   Considerable amounts of K^+ are secreted into the distal tubules. This K^+ is transported in the region of the tubule in a direction opposite to sodium (with the latter entering the cell) but not rigidly coupled with sodium. Either all or most K^+ movement is caused by the very negative electrical gradient created inside the cell when Na^+ is pumped out. The negativity pulls K^+ into the cell, which then diffuses out into the tubular lumen for excretion. (**Ref. 2,** pp. 650–654, 665)

76. (**C**)   Creatinine in not readily absorbed but rather is secreted in the proximal tubule to actually increase the excretion of creatinine by approximately 20%. (**Ref. 2,** pp. 650–652)

77. (**B**)   The ADH secreted from the hypothalamic-posterior pituitary system results in a decrease in urine output. This hormone also causes an increase in H_2O reabsorption from the collecting ducts (and to a slight extent from the distal tubules as well). The urine that is excreted is thus highly concentrated. (**Ref. 2,** pp. 650–658)

78. (**B**)   The action potential is characterized by an immediate voltage reduction and attains an amplitude of about 120 mV at its peak and is positive in polarity. This potential returns slowly to its original resting value after the occurrence of afterpotentials. (**Ref. 2,** pp. 45–51)

79. (**A**)   The ability of Na^+ to cross the membrane is almost immediate after the membrane resistance changes. The unit of membrane resistance is in ohms/cm^2. (**Ref. 2,** pp. 50–51)

80. (**C**)   After some delay (at peak of Na^+ conductance), the membrane reverses its permeability to favor K^+, and then is reflected by a K^+ conductance shape that demonstrates the delay and late onset. The K^+ conductance lasts until the membrane voltage is restored to its resting value. (**Ref. 2,** pp. 50–51)

81. (**A**)   The slow charging of the membrane as the stimulus current is applied leads to membrane depolarization that is nonpropagated (the response is localized and does not spread very far). (**Ref. 2,** pp. 50–51)

82. (**D**)   As the membrane potential repolarizes its rate, repolarization is slowed for a few milliseconds prior to reaching its resting level. This period is called the negative afterpotential and is believed to result from a K^+ accumulation just immediately outside the membrane. As a result, the concentration ratio of K^+ across the mem-

brane is a little less than normal, preventing the immediate return of the potential to its steady-state value. (**Ref. 2,** pp. 50–51)

83. (C) The overshoot represents the voltage above the zero level and is a result of excess Na^+ entering the cell. (**Ref. 2,** pp. 50–51

84. (B) The spike is a term used to designate the sudden, rapid nerve and muscle depolarization resulting from the Na^+ influx (and to some extent Ca^{2+} influx). (**Ref. 2,** pp. 50–51)

85. (E) When the excited membrane has repolarized to its resting level, the membrane potential may for a short period of time be a little more negative. This period of time is called the positive after-potential. It is the potential which occurs toward the end of repolarization and is more negative by just a few millivolts. It lasts for a few milliseconds in duration and may be the result of excess efflux pumping of the Na^+. (*t* is also a period of time during which the cell is in a less excitable state.) (**Ref. 2,** pp. 50–51)

86. (F) The threshold potential is that level of membrane voltage to which the membrane potential must be reduced before the Na^+ channels are all open and when the depolarization process becomes self-generative. (**Ref. 2,** pp. 50–51)

87. (G) At a certain point during the depolarization process a sufficient amount of Na^+ ion has entered the cell to exactly neutralize the negative potential. The potential inside the cell is equal to the potential outside the cell and, in fact, no potential or voltage gradient exists across the membrane. (**Ref. 2,** pp. 50–51)

2

Membrane, Neuromuscular, and Sensory Physiology

MULTIPLE CHOICE

DIRECTIONS (Questions 88–145): Each of the questions or incomplete statements below is followed by five suggested answers or completions. Select the **one** that is **best** in each case.

88. The "oscillatory" type of electrical activity recorded from visceral smooth muscle may be
    A. pacemaker potentials and initiated by Ca^{2+} influx
    B. pacemaker potentials and initiated by Cl^- influx
    C. pacemaker potentials and initiated by Na^+ influx
    D. local electronic change in potential not related to ionic movement
    E. pacemaker potential and initiated by K^+ influx

89. Sensory impulses arising in the periphery
    A. must all pass through the reticular formation
    B. never pass through the reticular formation
    C. they all pass through the reticular formation or may all bypass it depending on the modality
    D. pass in part through the reticular formation and in part bypass it
    E. ascend by unknown pathways to the cortex

90. Rapid adaptation of touch sensation is due to
   A. a decrease in firing rate despite continuous deformation of the receptor and/or return of the receptor to its original conformation despite continuous application of pressure
   B. maintenance of the distorted receptor conformation
   C. compensating mechanisms at the basal ganglia level
   D. failure of the cerebrum to detect a continuous sensory input
   E. failure of continuous sensory input to get through the reticular activating system

91. Visceral pain is most often due to
   A. electrical stimulation
   B. chemical stimulation
   C. stretch
   D. compression
   E. high body temperature

92. If you are placed in a chair and spun around from your left to right
   A. you will display left nystagmus
   B. you will display right nystagmus
   C. you will have your left semicircular canal maximally stimulated
   D. the pursuit phase will be to the left
   E. no nystagmus will occur

93. In certain pathologic conditions a sudden stretch of a skeletal muscle will result in sustained rhythmic contractions. This phenomenon is referred to as
   A. clonus
   B. hyperreflexia
   C. hyporeflexia
   D. spasticity
   E. clasp knife reflex

94. Receptors that mimic cholinergic receptors are called
   A. beta receptors
   B. serotinergic
   C. alpha receptors
   D. muscarinic
   E. dopaminergic

95. Which of the following is true with respect to the corticospinal pathway?
   A. It facilitates flexor motoneurons
   B. It is only a contralateral pathway
   C. It must be intact for a positive Babinski reflex
   D. It is an ipsilateral path at the level of the lower pons
   E. If it is severed at the level of the cerebral peduncles, primarily extrapyramidal effects will appear

96. As we are all aware, when we lift a load with our hands the load is not moved with sudden, jerky motion but rather via a smooth-graded motion. This situation arises because the muscle
   A. asynchronously recruits its individual motor units
   B. contracts all or none in a tetanic fashion
   C. adjusts its elastic components to the load to absorb some of the kinetic energy of the contraction and therefore to make it appear smooth
   D. neural impulse rate increases but number of units does not
   E. number of units for any muscle that fires is predetermined and constant

97. The auditory cortex is
   A. necessary for perception of temporal patterns of sound
   B. not necessary for understanding speech
   C. tonotopically organized
   D. represented by high frequencies in the anterior portion
   E. only found in the left hemisphere

98. "Stress relaxation" is a phenomenon seen in smooth muscle and allows organs lined by smooth muscle to act as reservoirs (e.g., spleen, uterus). The capability of smooth muscle to demonstrate this phenomenon is caused by a property called
   A. tonus
   B. tetanus
   C. tone
   D. plasticity
   E. paresis

99. The CNS receives and processes information from the periphery. Which of the following choices BEST describes a method of sensory input?

    A. The magnitude of a sensory stimulus is received by the CNS and interpreted by changes in action potential conduction velocities

    B. The magnitude of a sensory stimulus is received by the CNS and interpreted by a change in action potential amplitude

    C. The magnitude of a sensory stimulus is received by the CNS and interpreted by a change in action potential frequencies

    D. The magnitude of a sensory stimulus is received by the CNS and interpreted by a change in awareness not involving action potentials

    E. The magnitude of a sensory stimulus is received by the CNS and interpreted according to the divergence of the stimulus during transmission

100. Hyperkinetic syndromes, such as chorea and athetosis, are usually associated with pathologic changes in

    A. the motor areas of the cerebral cortex

    B. the pathways for recurrent collateral inhibition in the spinal cord

    C. those portions of the reticular formation controlling the gamma innervation of muscle spindles

    D. the anterior hypothalamus

    E. the basal ganglia complex

101. The terminology used to denote deep sensation is

    A. proprioception

    B. exteroception

    C. chemoreception

    D. interoreception

    E. nociception

102. Neuromuscular transmission
    A. is caused by the release of ACh from the muscle side of the junction
    B. shows a permeability change to Na^+ and K^+ at the receptor site during the endplate potential (EPP)
    C. may be facilitated by curare in myasthenia gravis
    D. is blocked by curare because it competes with the Na^+ entry during the muscle action potential
    E. is solely an electronic function

103. Two-point discrimination is
    A. most effective on the hands
    B. most effective on the legs
    C. most effective on the face
    D. least effective on the face
    E. most effective on the big toe

104. The Golgi tendon organ
    A. decreases activity during strong muscle contraction
    B. stops activity during strong muscle contraction
    C. is a muscle-length receptor
    D. is a muscle-tension receptor
    E. is a motor effector organ

105. The visual cortex has
    A. simple cells
    B. complex cells
    C. hypocomplex cells
    D. distance cells
    E. bipolar cells

106. The muscles of the middle ear
    A. are always fully contracted
    B. protect the cochlea from overstimulation
    C. are necessary for auditory sensation
    D. are reflexly activated by loud sounds
    E. are vestigial in function

107. The action potential in a pacinian corpuscle starts at the
    A. end of the non-myelinated fiber
    B. first node of Ranvier
    C. inside capsule layer

D. second node of Ranvier
E. outer capsule layer

108. The major cation directly involved in the isotonic contraction of skeletal muscle is
A. Na^+
B. Ca^+
C. K^+
D. Mg^{2+}
E. Cl^-

109. Contraction of muscles to hold the body upright against gravity depends largely on activity in the
A. spinal cord
B. cerebral cortex
C. reticular formation
D. hypothalamus
E. basal ganglia

110. Alpha motoneurons
A. supply the motor innervation for Golgi tendon organs
B. supply the motor innervation for the smooth muscle fibers
C. supply the motor innervation for muscle spindles
D. are the final common pathway for the motor system
E. supply the motor innervation for all glands

111. The generator potential of a receptor
A. is fixed in amplitude and unrelated to stimulus intensity
B. does not show degrees of adaptation
C. is responsible for frequency-modulated nerve discharge
D. is self-propagating and is nondecremental
E. is entirely chemical in nature

112. All of the following are true in regard to the strength-duration curve EXCEPT
A. it is a relationship between the duration of the stimulus and the amplitude of response
B. it has a rheobase which is two times chronaxie
C. cannot be characterized by its chronaxie
D. it differs for different tissue (i.e., nerve and muscle)
E. it is necessary to determine the decremented characteristics of a nerve

113. When light rays come to a focus behind the retina, the eye is said to be
    A. hypermetropic
    B. presbyopic
    C. astigmatic
    D. myopic
    E. emmetropic

114. For skeletal muscle one would expect an inverse relationship between
    A. muscle length and force of contraction
    B. load opposing contraction and velocity of contraction
    C. velocity of contraction (at low velocities) and efficiency of contraction
    D. muscle mass and cross-sectional area
    E. rest length and contracted length

115. A substance used experimentally to differentiate the endplate potential from the muscle action potential is
    A. epinephrine
    B. histamine
    C. norepinephrine
    D. tubocurarine
    E. acetylcholine

116. The red reaction of the triple response is a skin reaction which is
    A. due to a firm pressure with a pointed object
    B. observed as a red line across the line of pressure
    C. not dependent on nervous mechanism(s)
    D. bounded by white areas
    E. all are correct

117. The monosynaptic reflex (as in the myotatic reflex) is
    A. the result of spindle activation
    B. facilitated by stimulation of gamma motor efferents to the homonymous muscle
    C. excitatory to the homonymous muscle
    D. inhibitory to antagonistic muscles
    E. all are correct

118. The diffuse character of pain from the gastrointestinal tract is probably due to the
    A. diffuse nature of pathways in the central nervous system
    B. absence of a visual correlate for the experience
    C. absence of segmental arrangement of pain fibers from the viscera
    D. sparsity of pain fibers compared to cutaneous area
    E. A and C are correct

119. Reflex stepping
    A. does not require connections to the cerebellum
    B. is based primarily on unilateral cord reflexes
    C. does not occur if the plantar surface is prevented from touching the ground
    D. is probably modulated in the intact animal by group II fibers
    E. requires an intact spinal cord

120. Qualities of pain include
    A. pricking
    B. referred
    C. burning
    D. A and C are correct
    E. A, B, and C are correct

121. Myopia
    A. results when the image that is transmitted by the lens is in focus in front of the retina
    B. results when the image is behind the retina
    C. is corrected by a concave lens
    D. A and C are correct
    E. B and C are correct

122. The role of the parasympathetic nervous system in gastrointestinal motility is
    A. essential
    B. permissive
    C. unknown
    D. modulating
    E. A and D are correct

123. When smooth muscle is stretched within physiologic limits
   A. the tension that develops is because of elastic elements only
   B. the muscle contracts due to the depolarization
   C. the membrane repolarizes
   D. syncytial conduction is enhanced
   E. B and D are correct

124. The distribution pattern of body hair is determined by
   A. androgens in men but not in women
   B. sex
   C. sex and androgens
   D. heredity in women, androgens in men
   E. none of the above

125. The saccule
   A. contains hair cells
   B. signals information about the head in space
   C. signals information about linear acceleration
   D. has a macula containing sensory cells that are directionally specific
   E. A and C are correct

126. Summation of muscle contraction can occur by
   A. recruitment of more motor units
   B. recruitment of additional muscle groups
   C. A and B are correct
   D. muscle hypertrophy
   E. all are correct

127. Pain receptors never are
   A. free nerve endings
   B. widespread in superficial layers of skin
   C. widespread in arterial walls
   D. encapsulated receptors
   E. A, B, and C are correct

128. Glaucoma may be caused by
   A. obstruction in the angle of the anterior chamber
   B. obstruction at the pupil
   C. obstruction in the canal of Schlemm
   D. destruction of the ciliary secretory epithelium
   E. A, B, and C are correct

129. Which of the following include sensations carried in the dorsal columns?
     A. Joint sensation
     B. Discriminative touch and vibration
     C. A and B are correct
     D. Heat
     E. All are correct

130. During photopic vision, the
     A. cones contain pigment that is sensitive to a specific color
     B. rods are not stimulated
     C. cones are responsible for most color distinction
     D. visual acuity is lower than in scotopic vision
     E. A and C are correct

131. Pain control
     A. can occur by activating the analgesia system
     B. depends on an overstimulation of fibers
     C. may occur by inhibition of the somatosensory endings in the skin over the area of pain
     D. involves corticifugal signals
     E. A and C are correct

132. The clasp knife reflex
     A. is the result of stimulation of a multisynaptic pathway and may protect the muscle from overload
     B. is referred to as the inverse myotatic reflex
     C. contributes to the smooth onset and termination of contraction
     D. is caused by activation of the Golgi tendon organs and relaxes the muscle following contraction
     E. all are correct

133. In the auditory system
     A. the superior olive plays a major role in sound localization
     B. extensive bilateral representation exists as a result of crossing and recrossing of fibers
     C. there is multiplicity of tonotopic representation, each level comprising from two to five separate maps of the cochlea
     D. there is tonotopic organization
     E. A and C are correct

134. Visual acuity is greatest in
- **A.** an area that contains mostly rods
- **B.** the fovea centralis
- **C.** the lateral edges of the retina
- **D.** dark lighting conditions
- **E.** B and D are correct

135. Chorea is
- **A.** a constant, uncoordinated, random, uncontrolled flexing type of movement
- **B.** the result of a lesion of the motor cortex
- **C.** often seen in Huntington's disease
- **D.** found only bilaterally
- **E.** B and D are correct

136. The frequency of action potentials in the nerve fiber (impulse rate)
- **A.** is slower for receptor potentials at or just above the threshold and increases as the potential rises above threshold
- **B.** is proportional to the amplitude of the receptor potential
- **C.** A and B are correct
- **D.** is independent of the strength of the applied stimuli
- **E.** all are correct

137. Which of the following is true regarding physiologic optics?
- **A.** Accommodation or changes in refractive power is accomplished by changes in the shape of the lens
- **B.** Accommodation or changes in refractive power is accomplished by displacement of the lens relative to the retina
- **C.** The major refractive power of the eye resides in the cornea
- **D.** The major refractive power of the eye resides in the lens
- **E.** A, B, and C are correct

138. The dermatome rule is used
- **A.** clinically by physicians to determine levels of pain perception
- **B.** to explain referred pain
- **C.** to discern the slow pain response
- **D.** to determine the extent of cutaneous tissue damage
- **E.** A and C are correct

139. The influx of sodium ions into a muscle fiber by the actions of acetylcholine
   A. decreases membrane potentials (makes resting potential less negative)
   B. increases membrane potential (makes resting potential more negative)
   C. is voltage activated
   D. is current activated
   E. A and C are correct

140. At the termination of an action potential, the potential sometimes fails to return to the resting level for another few milliseconds. Which of the following may be said regarding this phenomenon?
   A. Termed the positive after potential
   B. Most likely to occur after a series of rapidly repeated action potential
   C. Results from the excessive permeability of potassium ions
   D. Results from the build-up of sodium ions within the cell
   E. B and D are correct

141. The velocity of conduction in nerve fibers
   A. is roughly 0.5 m/s in unmyelinated fibers
   B. is as high as 10,000 m/s in myelinated fibers
   C. decreases with the diameter in myelinated fibers
   D. increases directly with the diameter in unmyelinated fibers
   E. B and D are correct

142. Unilateral labyrinthectomy at the midpontine level causes
   A. spasticity of limb muscles on the side of the lesion
   B. a loss of all postural reflexes that have their centers in the medulla
   C. hyperextension of contralateral link
   D. no spontaneous nystagmus
   E. A and C are correct

143. In non-active nerve fibers in the body
   A. net efflux of sodium is greater than net influx of sodium
   B. passive diffusion of potassium outward is greater than passive diffusion of potassium inward
   C. passive diffusion of sodium inward equals the passive diffusion of potassium outward
   D. passive diffusion of sodium inward equals active transport of sodium outward
   E. B and D are correct

144. Depolarization of the neuromuscular junction is
   A. caused by nicotine
   B. caused by acetylcholine (ACh)
   C. A and B are correct
   D. blocked by atropine
   E. all are correct

145. The optic axis of the eye
   A. is the same as the visual axis
   B. passes through the nodal point
   C. is the axis along which the eye is directed
   D. is the axis of optical symmetry
   E. B and D are correct

MATCHING

DIRECTIONS (Questions 146–150): The following group of questions consists of a set of lettered components, followed by a list of numbered words or phrases. For **each** numbered word or phrase, select the **one** lettered component that is most closely associated with it. Each lettered component may be selected once, more than once, or not at all.

   A. tonic neck reflexes
   B. optical righting reaction
   C. muscle spindle reflexes
   D. tonic labyrinthine reflexes
   E. crossed extensor

146. Is necessary for withdrawal reaction

147. Initiates contraction after rapid extension

148. When head turns to left, left foreleg extends

149. When neck is dorsiflexed, forelegs extend

150. After section of cranial nerve VIII the head can still be properly oriented

---

DIRECTIONS (Questions 151–169): Each group of questions below consists of a diagram with lettered components followed by a list of numbered words or phrases. For **each** numbered word or phrase, select the **one** lettered component that is most closely associated with it. Each lettered component may be selected once, more than once, or not at all.

Questions 151–154 (Figure 8):

151. indicates the total muscle tension

152. indicates the resting length

153. indicates the tension developed by the passive elements

154. indicates the active tension developed by the contractile elements

Questions 155–158 (Figure 9):

155. indicates the rheobase

156. indicates the chronaxie

157. indicates the utilization time

158. indicates the strength-duration relationship

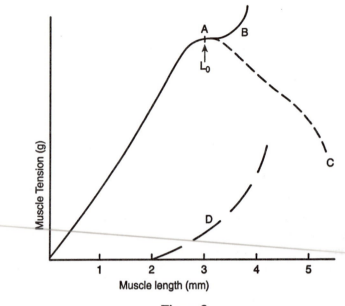

Figure 8

Figure 9

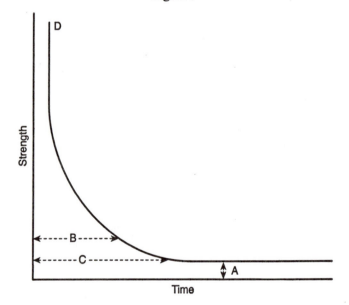

Question 159 (Figure 10):

159. the relationship between K^+ concentration and membrane voltage in living cells

Questions 160–169 (Figure 11):

160. the direction of K^+ flux during repolarization

161. the direction of Na^+ flux during depolarization

162. the direction of impulse propagation (orthograde)

163. the voltage gradient across the resting membrane

164. the voltage gradient across the membrane during activity

165. the fluid containing more K^+ (at rest)

166. the fluid containing more Cl^- (at rest)

Figure 10

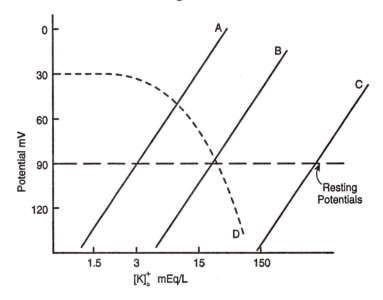

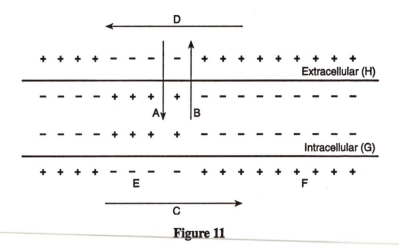

Figure 11

167. the fluid containing more protein⁻ (at rest)

168. the fluid containing more Na⁺ (at rest)

169. would indicate retrograde propagation

Membrane, Neuromuscular, and Sensory Physiology

Answers and Discussion

88. (A) The instability of the membrane, its tendency for spontaneous depolarization in visceral muscle, may be related to the fact that the smooth muscle membrane has more voltage-gated calcium channels than sodium channels. The flow of calcium into the interior of the fiber is responsible for the slow action potentials of smooth muscle. (**Ref. 2,** pp. 71–74)

89. (D) It is a general rule of the nervous system that sensory impulses arising in a primary sensory neuron are distributed by way of collaterals, projection tracts, and secondary relays to widely separated parts of the nervous system. This is true of the reticular system as well, since sensory impulses partly pass through it and partly bypass it. (**Ref. 1,** pp. 122–132ff)

90. (A) The corpuscular structure of the pacinian corpuscle rapidly adapts to the deformation of the tissue because fluid within the capsule redistributes itself so that the pressure becomes essentially equal, thus reducing the receptor potential. (**Ref. 2,** pp. 106–108)

91. (C) Stretch due to distension is the most common cause of visceral pain. (**Ref. 2,** pp. 126–131)

92. (A) The ocular movements are in the same direction as the convection hydraulic current set up in the semicircular canals. The nystagmus consists of a slow (pursuit) and a fast (saccadic) movement, and it is named in accordance with the direction of the fast movement. The slow movement is toward the side stimulated. Thus, one would display left nystagmus. (**Ref. 2,** pp. 150–151)

93. (A) Clonus is the name used to describe regular rhythmic contractions of a skeletal muscle in situ under sustained stretch. (**Ref. 2,** pp. 65–67)

94. (D) Acetylcholine activates at least two different types of receptors. These are called muscarinic and nicotinic receptors. (**Ref. 2,** pp. 88–89)

95. (A) Flexor motoneurons are predominantly facilitated by the corticospinal pathway. (**Ref. 2,** pp. 185–187)

96. (A) Special neurogenic mechanisms in the spinal cord normally increase both the impulse rate and the number of motor units firing at the same time. The tension exerted by the whole muscle is still continuous and non-jerky because the different motor units fire asynchronously. (**Ref. 2,** pp. 62–67)

97. (C) Certain parts of the primary auditory cortex are known to respond to high frequencies and other parts to low frequencies. In monkeys, the posterior part of the supratemporal plane responds to high frequencies, while the anterior part responds to low frequencies. Thus, discrete tones are localized in discrete regions of the auditory cortex. (**Ref. 2,** p. 163–164)

98. (D) A very important characteristic of smooth muscle is its ability to change length greatly without marked changes in tension. This results from fiber rearrangement due to smooth muscle plasticity. (**Ref. 2,** pp. 71–74)

99. (C) The frequency of action potentials in the nerve fiber (impulse rate) is almost directly proportional to the amplitude of the receptor potential. (**Ref. 2,** pp. 113–121)

100. (E) Chorea is associated with degeneration of the caudate nucleus; athetosis is caused by lesions in the lenticular nucleus. **(Ref. 2, p. 196)**

101. (A) Events in the external and internal environments are first detected by receptors that can be categorized according to where the input is initiated: exteroceptors in the skin, proprioceptors in deep tissue (muscles, tendons, and joints). **(Ref. 2, pp. 126–131)**

102. (B) The amplitude of the action potential at the neuromuscular junction depends on permeability changes to Na^+ and K^+ at the receptor site during the EPP. **(Ref. 2, pp. 75–88)**

103. (A) Two-point discrimination consists of two needles pressed against the skin, and the subject determines whether he feels two points of stimulation or one point. On the tips of the fingers, a person can distinguish two separate points even when the needles are as close together as 2 mm. **(Ref. 2, pp. 123–125)**

104. (E) The Golgi tendon organ detects tension applied to the tendon by muscle contraction. The signal from the tendon organ supposedly excites inhibitory interneurons and these, in turn, inhibit the alpha mononeurons to the respective muscle. **(Ref. 2, pp. 116–117)**

105. (B) The majority of neurons in the striate cortex and all of them in extrastriate cortex possess receptive fields that are more elaborately organized than those of simple cells. Complex neurons are found in all cortical layers. They respond optimally to a properly oriented slit, edge, or dark bar, and for any one neuron certain spatial patterns are more effective than others. **(Ref. 1, pp. 653, 725 ff)**

106. (D) When loud sounds are transmitted through the ossicular system into the central nervous system a reflex occurs after a latent period of only 50 msec to cause contractions of both the stapedius and tensor tympani muscles. This attenuation reflex can reduce the intensity of sound transmission by as much as 30 to 40 dB. **(Ref. 2, pp. 154–162)**

107. (B) Deformation of the capsule causes a sudden change in the membrane potential by increasing its permeability and allowing positively charged sodium ions to leak to the interior of the fiber. This change in local potential causes a local circuit of current flow that spreads along the nerve fiber to its myelinated portion. At the first node of Ranvier the local current flow initiates action potentials in the nerve fiber. (**Ref. 2,** pp. 106–107)

108. **(B)** Evidence suggests that excitation–contraction coupling is effected simply by release of Ca^{2+} from the sarcoplasmic reticulum. The subsequent translocation of Ca^{2+} to troponin with consequent activation of actomyosin ATPase results in association of actin and myosin when the Ca^{2+} concentration has been raised sufficiently. (**Ref. 2,** pp. 59–61)

109. **(C)** When a person or an animal is in a standing position continuous impulses are transmitted from the reticular formation into the spinal cord and then to extensor muscles to stiffen the limbs. (**Ref. 2,** pp. 184–194)

110. **(D)** The alpha motoneurons give rise to large type-A alpha nerve fibers that innervate the skeletal muscles. They are the final common pathway for any motor response. (**Ref. 2,** pp. 113–119)

111. **(C)** In all sensory receptors, the amplitude of the generator potential increases as the strength of the stimulus increases, but the additional response usually becomes progressively less as the strength of stimulus becomes great. (**Ref. 2,** pp. 107–108)

112. **(E)** The least possible voltage at which a nerve will fire is called the rheobase, and the time required for this least voltage to stimulate the fiber is called the utilization time. If the voltage is increased to twice the rheobase voltage, the time to stimulate the fiber is called the chronaxie and is a means of expressing the excitability of different tissues. (**Ref. 2,** pp. 52–53)

113. **(A)** When the axial length of an eye is too short relative to its focal length, the retina will intercept the bundle of rays from a distant object before it comes to a focus. A person with this kind of defect is said to be hypermetropic. (**Ref. 2,** pp. 138–140)

114. **(B)** A decreasing velocity of a skeletal muscle seems to be caused mainly by the fact that a load on a contracting muscle is a reverse force that opposes the contractile force caused by muscle contraction. Therefore, the net force that is available to cause velocity of shortening is correspondingly reduced. (**Ref. 2,** pp. 62–64)

115. **(D)**   The endplate potential and the action potential may be separated by utilizing d-tubocurarine, which inhibits and reduces the postsynaptic depolarizing action of ACh. (**Ref. 2,** pp. 84–89)

116. **(E)**   The red reaction to the triple response is the reaction to a firm stimulus of a pointed object over the skin area. The compress is a red boil (local red line due to venular dilation) with a pale area (on either side due to capillary constriction). This is not dependent upon nervous mechanisms since it can occur after autonomic nerve section and degeneration. (**Ref. 2,** p. 570)

117. **(E)**   The muscle spindle reflex originates in the muscle spindle whereby a type-IA nerve fiber enters the dorsal root of the spinal cord and synapses directly with an anterior motoneuron, which transmits an appropriate reflex signal back to the same muscle. This results in its contraction. All the factors listed occur in this reflex. (**Ref. 2,** pp. 113–116)

118. **(D)**   The diffuse nature of visceral pain is established by the relatively light innervation of the area. (**Ref. 2,** pp. 126–131)

119. **(C)**   If a well-heated spinal animal is held up from the table, and its legs allowed to fall downward, the stretch in the limbs occasionally elicits stepping reflexes that involve all four limbs. (**Ref. 2,** pp. 189–193)

120. **(D)**   Pain has been classified into three different types: pricking, burning, and aching pain. (**Ref. 2,** pp. 126–131)

121. **(D)**   Myopia is a condition in which the image of a distant object is formed not on the retina but in front of it. In myopia, some of the excessive refractive power can be neutralized by placing a concave spherical lens in front of the eye that will diverge rays. (**Ref. 2,** pp. 137–140)

122. **(D)**   The parasympathetic division releases acetylcholine and catecholamines which affect the frequency of spike discharge. This system does not initiate activity, but merely modifies or modulates an existing activity of the gastrointestinal system. (**Ref. 2,** pp. 203–207)

123. (B) Stretch is the most common physiologic stimulus for smooth muscle depolarization leading to contraction. (**Ref. 2, pp. 71–74**)

124. (C) The genetic layout that will impart the characteristics of an individual plus the presence and exposure to androgens required for hair distribution determine the distribution of hair. (**Ref. 2, pp. 395–398**)

125. (E) Located on the wall of both the utriculus and saccule is a small area slightly more than 2 mm in diameter called a macula. Each macula is a sensory area for detecting the orientation of the head with respect to the direction of gravitational pull or of other acceleratory forces. Each macula is covered by a gelatinous layer in which many small calcium carbonate crystals, called otoconia, are embedded. Also in the macula are thousands of hair cells which project cilia into the gelatinous layer. Around the bases of the hair cells are intwined sensory axons of the vestibular nerve. (**Ref. 2, pp. 154–156**)

126. (C) The stimulation of more motor units, increasing rate of stimulation, and recruitment of additional muscle groups will increase motive force. Hypertrophy associated with exercise will allow a greater total force. (**Ref. 2, pp. 61–67**)

127. (D) Pain receptors are not encapsulated, are not easily adaptive, and respond to tissue damage, heat, and ischemia. (**Ref. 2, pp. 126–128**)

128. (E) Glaucoma is a disease of the eye in which intraocular pressure becomes pathologically high. In nearly all cases of glaucoma, the abnormally high pressure results from increased resistance to fluid outflow at the iridocorneal junction. The aqueous humor is produced by the ciliary secretory epithelium so its destruction should cause intraocular pressure to decrease. (**Ref. 2, p. 133**)

129. (C) On entering the central nervous system, the thermal fibers travel in the lateral spinothalamic tract. Joint and muscle sensation and discriminatory touch are carried in the dorsal column. (**Ref. 2, pp. 122–123**)

130. **(E)** Color vision is mediated primarily by the cones which contain three pigments sensitive to blue, green, and red. (**Ref. 2,** pp. 147–153)

131. **(A)** By stimulation of large sensory neural fibers the mechanoreceptor sensory afferents can suppress pain signals. Also the analgesia system can block pain at the initial entry point to the spinal cord. (**Ref. 2,** pp. 130–132)

132. **(E)** In a spinal animal, the tendon reflexes that regulate tension are hyperactive and clonus occurs; sustained stretch reflexes are observed. This inverse myotatic reflex is a lengthening or clasp knife phenomenon and follows the four factors listed. (**Ref. 2,** pp, 189–191)

133. **(A)** Simple hearing functions such as threshold sensitivity, recognition of pure tones, frequency discrimination, and intensity discrimination are not severely impaired by rather large experimental lesions of central auditory structures. (**Ref. 2,** pp.163–164)

134. **(B)** The fovea centralis in the center of the macula is best able to distinguish visual stimuli. This area is made up almost entirely of cones and requires higher light intensities for effective function. (**Ref. 2,** pp. 133–135)

135. **(E)** The cardinal criteria for the diagnosis of Huntington's disease are choreoathetoid hyperkinesis and hereditary disposition characterized by flicking movements which become more severe with time. (**Ref. 2,** p. 196)

136. **(C)** When a stimulus, such as pressure, is applied to a receptor, the receptor fires at a rate that is proportional to the applied pressure. Those impulses that result in action potentials with takeoff potentials at or near the firing threshold generally have greater action potential amplitudes and, therefore, are lower in frequency. As the frequency increases the action potential amplitude decreases. (**Ref. 2,** pp. 107–108)

137. **(E)** The cornea is responsible for most of the refractory power of the eye (43 diopters); however, this is fixed. The lens has less power but can adjust (13 to 26 diopters). Accommodation is accomplished by changes in the shape of the lens, with some displacement of the lens relative to the retina. (**Ref. 2,** pp. 137–139

138. **(B)** Referred pain is the perception of visceral pain as emanating from a cutaneous area of healthy tissue. The explanation of this phenomenon is that the area in which the pain is felt is innervated by neurons from the same spinal segment innervating the affected organ. (**Ref. 2,** p. 129)

139. **(A)** Excitation of a skeletal muscle fiber by the action of acetylcholine results in a ligand-activated influx of sodium ions. This results in an increase in the positive direction of the local membrane potential. (**Ref. 2,** p. 59)

140. **(B)** Rapidly repeated action potential results in a build-up of potassium ions on the outside surface of the cell. This delays the return of the potential to resting level values. This is termed negative afterpotential. (**Ref. 2,** pp. 46–47)

141. **(A)** For unmyelinated fibers, the velocity increases with the square root of the fiber diameter and directly with diameter in myelinated fibers. (**Ref. 2,** pp. 52–54)

142. **(E)** Unilateral labyrinthectomy results in limb rigidity in the side of the lesion and hyperextension and increased tendon reflexes in the contralateral limbs. (**Ref. 2,** p. 166)

143. **(E)** A normal nerve at rest (non-active) has a membrane potential of about -90 mV. This is maintained by the active transport system of the coupled Na^+–K^+ pump. Thus, the normal passive diffusion of Na^+ inward is counterbalanced by the active outward transport of Na^+. The normally greater outward diffusion of K^+ is balanced by the pumping of K^+ back into the cell. (**Ref. 2,** pp. 45–51)

144. **(C)** The neuromuscular junction contains nicotinic cholinergic receptors. They are stimulated by nicotine and ACh and inhibited by curare. (**Ref. 2,** pp. 101–104)

145. **(C)** The optic axis is different from the visual axis. Though they both pass through the nodal point, the visual axis is the line

along which the eye is directed while the optic axis includes a line that runs through the center of the cornea, pupil, and lens. (**Ref. 2,** pp. 137–140)

146. (**E**)   Crossed extensor reflex facilitates support of the body by the contralateral side when a nociceptive withdrawal response is elicited. (**Ref. 2,** p. 119)

147. (**C**)   When a muscle is stretched, muscle spindles are activated which reflexly causes contraction of the same muscle. This is the basis of the stretch reflex. (**Ref. 2,** pp. 113–118)

148. (**A**)   Input from tonic neck receptors has a major effect on tone in the forelimbs. (**Ref. 2,** pp. 116–121)

149. (**D**)   The tonically active receptors of the labyrinth affect forelimb tone through the intermediate of neck muscle tone. (**Ref. 2,** pp. 116–121)

150. (**B**)   The visual system plays the most prominent role in righting reflexes. (**Ref. 2,** pp. 188–191)

151. (**B**)   The total muscle tension represents the tension being contributed by both the active and passive elements and, therefore, will continue and increase as the length is increased. (**Ref. 2,** pp. 62–63)

152. (**A**)   The resting length, or L_0, is the muscle length that is set in the body and represents the maximal overlap between the actin and myosin. Therefore it will produce a drop in tension from that obtained at L_0. (**Ref. 2,** pp. 62–63)

153. (**D**)   The tension developed by the passive elements is the result of stretching of these elements, which behave like stretching a rubber band. Such tension therefore will continue to increase as stretch increases until all elements are broken. (**Ref. 2,** pp. 62–63)

154. (**C**)   The actin-myosin components yield the true muscle tension, and this tension is maximal at L_0. It may be obtained by subtracting the passive element tensions from the total muscle tension. (**Ref. 2,** pp. 62–63)

155. (A) The rheobase is a voltage that is sufficient in strength to evoke a response when the duration of the stimulus is permitted to last for a long time, even infinitely if necessary.

156. (B) Chronaxie is the time that it takes to evoke a membrane response when the strength of the stimulus is set at twice the rheobasic value.

157. (C) When the stimulus is permitted to flow for a long period of time, even to infinity (to ascertain the rheobase current), there will be a response (at the rheobase strength) called the utilization time.

158. (D) The slope of a strength-duration curve is exponential, and the parameters are inversely related.

159. (A) At a normal resting potential of about -90 mV, the $[K_o]$ is about 3 mEq/L. Increasing the $[K_o]$ will depolarize the membrane. Such changes do not occur when the Na^+ and Cl^- concentrations are altered. (**Ref. 2,** pp. 50–51)

160. (B); 161. (A); 162. (D); 163. (F); 164. (E); 165. (G); 166. (H); 167. (G); 168. (H); 169. (C) An impulse is essentially a series of currents flowing in and out of the cell membrane. Action potentials leave the membrane ahead of the region of depolarization and act as a cathode (current flow into a cathodal electrode). The action potential current acts on the membrane ahead of it. At this time the membrane permeability is such that Na^+ can move inside while the area behind it is repolarizing and K^+ ion flux is outward. As thus defined, the impulse in the figure is propagating from right to left (i.e., arrow D). At rest, the voltage gradient is positive outside and negative inside the cell with the concentration of Na^+ and Cl^- greater with extracellular fluid, while K^+ and anion protein molecule concentrations are greater in the intracellular fluid. (**Ref. 2,** pp. 47–51)

3

CNS Physiology

MULTIPLE CHOICE

DIRECTIONS: Each of the questions or incomplete statements below is followed by five suggested answers or completions. Select the **one** that is **best** in each case.

---

170. The capacity to display rage
   A. is eliminated when the cerebral cortex is removed
   B. is due to an imbalance of activity in large and small fibers
   C. is not affected by removal of the hypothalamus
   D. does not require any structure above the level of the hypothalamus
   E. is the major function of the ANS

171. The decrease in magnitude of a generator potential during sustained stimulation is called
   A. receptor perturbation
   B. adaptation
   C. refractoriness
   D. accommodation
   E. chronaxie

172. Normal blood flow to the brain is
A. greatly modified by vasomotor control
B. increased by high oxygen level
C. about 150 mL/min
D. about 750 mL/min
E. greatly increased during exercise

173. Synaptic innervation of a number of cells by one fiber is an example of
A. convergence
B. chronaxie
C. rheobase
D. divergence
E. reverberation

174. Activation of regional areas of the cortex
A. is accomplished by the reticular activating system
B. is accomplished by the diffuse thalamocortical system
C. is induced only by painful stimuli
D. may be associated with the direction of our attention to one area of our environment
E. is determined solely by blood flow

175. Fever due to infection is the result of
A. increased heat production followed by decreased heat loss
B. decreased heat loss followed by increased heat production
C. an action of bacterial pyrogens independent of the body's heat control mechanism
D. a functional hyperthyroidism caused by irritation of the thyroid and release of colloid
E. increased respiratory work

176. The vomiting center is located in the
A. cerebral cortex
B. thalamus
C. hypothalamus
D. medulla oblongata
E. cervical spinal cord

177. The inhibitory synaptic potential recorded from the cell body of a CNS neuron
   A. cannot be summed either temporally or spatially
   B. involves a selective increase in the permeability to K^+ and Cl^-
   C. cannot be opposed by stimulation of excitatory presynaptic neurons
   D. is not a normal occurrence during spinal reflex activity
   E. involves a selective increase in Ca^{2+} permeability

178. During the excitation of a nerve cell the peak of potassium efflux occurs
   A. after the spike and before the peak sodium influx
   B. before the spike and after the peak sodium influx
   C. before both spike and peak sodium influx
   D. after both spike and peak sodium influx
   E. coincident with the peak of sodium influx

179. The body temperature range that can be tolerated best during hypothermic cooling is (in °F)
   A. under 69°
   B. 70°–74°
   C. 75°–79°
   D. 80°–84°
   E. 85°–90°

180. The primary motor cortex
   A. receives no sensory input
   B. is active in the adjustment of motor activity to current sensory input
   C. is not necessary for fine motor movement
   D. gives rise to the extrapyramidal tract
   E. is localized only in the frontal lobe

181. Norepinephrine is probably the
   A. inhibitory transmitter at the alpha motoneuron
   B. excitatory transmitter acting on Renshaw cells
   C. transmitter at muscarinic synapses
   D. transmitter released from most postganglionic sympathetic fibers
   E. transmitter released from Purkinje cell synapses

182. The sympathetic division of the autonomic nervous system is characterized by
   A. presynaptic inhibition
   B. thoracolumbar outflow from the spinal cord
   C. short postganglionic fibers
   D. adrenergic preganglionic fibers
   E. the vagus nerve, which is its major component

183. Premotor cortex refers to
   A. some areas anterior to the primary motor cortex that can cause complex coordinate movements, such as speech, eye, and head movements
   B. an area of the motor cortex that is vital for the initiation of voluntary motor movements
   C. an area found in the temporal cortex that when stimulated allows the most primitive movements to take place
   D. a term often used to refer to the cerebellar cortex
   E. an area of the cortex in the vicinity of the insula

184. The motor cortex
   A. could be considered as six separate motor areas that when stimulated are especially likely to cause contraction of specific muscles
   B. can be considered to be composed of only small neurons
   C. is composed of primary motor, supplementary motor, somatic sensorimotor I, and somatic sensorimotor II areas
   D. can be found completely in the frontal lobe
   E. has no apparent organization of motor functions

185. The human rectal temperature at which permanent cell damage might result if it is prolonged is (in °F)
   A. 99°
   B. 101°
   C. 103°
   D. no effect is observed even at 110°
   E. 106°

186. The release of transmitter from nerve terminals into the synaptic cleft
   A. decreases dramatically when the nerve terminals are depolarized
   B. is associated with the influx of Ca^{2+} into the presynaptic membrane during an action potential in the nerve endings

    C. in a normal individual will always mise the postjunctional
       membrane above threshold if an action potential invades the
       nerve terminal
    D. is inhibited if the nerve terminals are hyperpolarized
    E. is an all-or-none phenomenon

187. Activation of various portions of the reticular formation
    A. can increase reflex activity
    B. can cause a complex motor movement such as speech
    C. can decrease reflex activity
    D. cannot affect the reflex activity
    E. acts to modulate reflex activity in conjunction with other
       brain structures

188. The condition known as REM (rapid eye movement) sleep is
    A. that point at which the individual becomes aware and alert
    B. characterized by slow high-voltage regular EEG activity
    C. referred to as paradoxical sleep
    D. related to EEG patterns seen in comatose patients
    E. characterized by total lack of all muscular activity

189. The cerebellum
    A. has a totally inhibitory output from its cortex
    B. has an excitatory output from its deep nuclear layers
    C. receives cortical input from mossy and climbing fibers
    D. has the same arrangement of cells as in most of the cerebellar
       cortex
    E. has a conscious interpretation of motor activity

190. A pair of electrodes placed on the surface of an uninjured nerve
    will record (following nerve stimulation)
    A. a resting potential followed by a monophasic compound
       action potential
    B. a zero potential followed by a diphasic compound action
       potential
    C. a zero potential followed by a monophasic compound action
       potential
    D. a resting potential followed by a diphasic compound action
       potential
    E. no potential change at all

191. At the postsynaptic membrane the EPSP is
  A. produced by ACh, giving rise to an increased permeability first to Na^+ and then after a delay to K^+
  B. produced by ACh, causing an increased permeability to Na^+ and K^+ simultaneously
  C. caused by a permeability increase to all ions except Na^+
  D. brought about by the splitting of ACh
  E. produced by ACh, giving rise initially to an increased K^+ permeability and then after a delay to Na^+

192. Metabolism in the nerve fiber
  A. supplies ATP to the sodium pump
  B. is blocked by cyanide or dinitrophenol with a directly correlated fall in resting and action potentials
  C. does not supply energy for fast transport of material
  D. controls the ACh level and, thus, the action potential
  E. is determined by its position in a nerve bundle

193. The cerebellum
  A. is associated with very rapid motor activity
  B. may be a timing device for measuring duration of rapid motor activity
  C. receives input from most of the cerebral cortex
  D. is only activated by painful stimuli
  E. is only associated with unlearned motor movements

194. Gamma-aminobutyric acid (GABA)
  A. hyperpolarizes motoneurons and is inhibitory in nature
  B. is blocked by strychnine
  C. is blocked by glycine
  D. probably is responsible for the inhibitory postsynaptic potential (IPSP) in alpha motoneurons
  E. is excitatory in nature

195. Alpha receptors differ from beta receptors in that
  A. alpha receptors are generally inhibitory, while the beta receptors are generally excitatory
  B. norepinephrine interacts with alpha receptors but not with beta receptors

C. alpha stimulation is generally followed by prolonged desensitization of the effector structures

D. alpha receptors are found only in glands

E. they allow an affinity of a hormone to a given organ

196. Blood pressure and the blood supply to various organs are in part regulated by variation in the caliber of the small blood vessels and controlled by a medullary center under the influence of

A. blood pressure changes detected by baroreceptors widely distributed along the great vessels and in the viscera

B. chemical changes in the blood

C. impulses from higher areas by which emotional activities are integrated

D. white blood cell concentrations in the blood

E. A, B, and C are correct

197. With regard to the "eating centers," they are

A. served by glucose receptors in the cells of the hypothalamus

B. not necessary for normal food intake

C. found in the medulla

D. stimulated by a satiety center

E. A and C are correct

198. Presynaptic inhibition depends on

A. reduced action potential amplitude

B. reduced transmitter release

C. A and B are correct

D. increased postsynaptic potential

E. all are correct

199. Experimentally induced depolarization of excitable membranes has revealed the following regarding membrane excitation

A. excitation is decreased at the anode

B. excitable membranes have no well-defined threshold

C. depolarization is caused by inward current in the membrane

D. depolarization is the result of a release of acetylcholine (ACh) in the membrane

E. A and C are correct

200. Spinal shock
  A. is produced by complete spinal transection
  B. is characterized by arc reflexes immediately after transection
  C. duration is often several weeks in humans
  D. is followed by spasticity
  E. all are correct

201. The major difference between grand mal epilepsy and psychomotor epilepsy is that in a psychomotor seizure there
  A. are myoclonic jerks
  B. is no massive convulsion
  C. is no postictal state
  D. is no aura
  E. A and C are correct

202. With a lateral quadrant lesion of the spinal cord, one may observe
  A. contralateral anesthesia
  B. contralateral hypothermia
  C. paresis, hyperreflexia, hypertonia ipsilaterally
  D. ipsilateral Babinski response
  E. all are correct

203. The thalamic syndrome includes
  A. emotional changes
  B. various degrees of anesthesia
  C. motor symptoms
  D. increased threshold to various stimuli
  E. A, B, and C are correct

204. Epilepsy
  A. is more likely to occur in females
  B. is a disorder of the CNS resulting from paroxysmal cerebral dysrhythmias
  C. is most often seen after 30 years of age
  D. cannot be produced by brain injuries
  E. A and B are correct

205. Sleep and wakefulness are related to which of the following structures?
  A. The intralaminar nuclei of the thalamus
  B. The posterior nucleus of the hypothalamus

    C. The periaqueductal gray
    D. The reticular formation
    E. All are correct

206. A pituitary adenoma might result in a variety of symptoms (dependent upon the tumor or growth), including
    A. amenorrhea
    B. diabetes insipidus
    C. bitemporal hemianopsia
    D. loss of adrenal function
    E. A, B, and C are correct

207. Clinical symptom(s) of cerebellar damage include
    A. adiadokokinesis
    B. asynergia
    C. ataxia
    D. intention tremor
    E. all are correct

208. The following physiologic responses are qualitatively common to both stimulation of the sympathetic nervous system and/or systemic administration of atropine
    A. bronchiolar dilation
    B. intestinal contraction
    C. increase in ventricular inotropicity
    D. increased secretion of sweat glands
    E. A, B, and C are correct

209. Which of the following is common to both excitatory postsynaptic potentials (EPSPs) and inhibitory postsynaptic potentials (IPSPs)?
    A. Spatial summation
    B. Temporal summation
    C. A and B are correct
    D. Alteration in Ca^{2+} concentration in the cell
    E. All are correct

210. Cortical-evoked potentials
  - **A.** are the electrical responses recorded following direct stimulation of either sense organs or afferent fibers that project to the area of cortex under study
  - **B.** is another term for electroencephalograph (EEG) activity
  - **C.** are those responses evoked by direct cortical stimulation
  - **D.** are the synchronized recordings after any thalamic stimulation
  - **E.** A and C are correct

211. Regarding cerebellar cortex function
  - **A.** after lesions, disturbances are contralateral to the lesion
  - **B.** it coordinates somatic motor activity and regulates muscle tone
  - **C.** sensory information received by the cerebellum is acted upon at a conscious level by this structure
  - **D.** speech is rarely disrupted after cerebellar damage
  - **E.** all are correct

212. Regarding sleep and wake mechanisms
  - **A.** the locus coeruleus initiates phasic desynchronization from the deep sleep pattern
  - **B.** lesions of the raphe system induce insomnia
  - **C.** pCO activity is induced by release of a pontine catecholamine pacemaker from inhibition
  - **D.** decreased release of serotonin results in an active hypersomnia
  - **E.** A, B, and C are correct

213. In spinal shock
  - **A.** the duration is a function of cerebral dominance
  - **B.** bladder function is lost
  - **C.** A and B are correct
  - **D.** noxious stimuli applied to the skin after spinal transection evoke flexion responses immediately
  - **E.** all are correct

214. Sweat glands are innervated by
  - **A.** cholinergic parasympathetic preganglionic fibers
  - **B.** cholinergic sympathetic postganglionic fibers
  - **C.** adrenergic sympathetic postganglionic fibers
  - **D.** cholinergic parasympathetic postganglionic fibers
  - **E.** none are correct

215. Clinical evaluation of the peripheral nerves of some alcoholics or vitamin B_1-deficient patients would reveal impairment of
   A. small myelinated fibers
   B. large myelinated fibers
   C. axolemma but not myelin
   D. touch, pressure, vibration, and position sense
   E. B and D are correct

216. The following has(have) been contemplated as the cause(s) of the epileptic foci of neurons
   A. postsynaptic excitation is increased
   B. astrocytes form scar tissue
   C. the amount of neurotransmitter released is deterred
   D. the neuronal membrane permeability to ions is changed
   E. all are correct

217. Stimulation of the parasympathetic nervous system causes
   A. accommodation for distant vision
   B. decreased glandular secretions
   C. myosis
   D. decreased HCl secretion in the stomach
   E. C and D are correct

218. Inhibition of fear and loss of emotion are prominent signs after lesion of
   A. mammillary bodies
   B. amygdaloid nuclei and limbic system
   C. cerebral frontal lobes
   D. cerebral motor cortex
   E. none are correct

219. Which of the following statements are true about Purkinje cells?
   A. They give rise to the only axons leaving the cerebellar cortex
   B. These cells are intermittently active
   C. They are always excitatory influences on the deep cerebellar nuclei
   D. They are the smallest cells of the cerebellum
   E. All are correct

220. Which of the following is characteristic of chemical synapses?
   A. Synaptic delay
   B. One-way conduction
   C. Susceptibility to drugs
   D. Summate algebraically
   E. All are correct

221. The action potential of a nerve membrane
   A. is followed after a delay by an inward movement of K^+
   B. has a reversal potential of about +85 mV
   C. has as its first active change an inward movement of Na^+
   D. has an inward movement of K^+ on its upward part
   E. B and D are correct

222. Paradoxical sleep
   A. usually occurs periodically during a night's sleep
   B. is usually associated with dreaming
   C. consists of abnormal sleep patterns
   D. is associated with increased muscle tone
   E. A and C are correct

223. Alpha and beta receptors are
   A. differentiated by blockade by atropine and curare
   B. differentiated on the basis of different sensitivities to norepinephrine and strychnine
   C. adrenergic receptors
   D. cholinergic receptors
   E. A and C are correct

224. The "all-or-none" law applies to which of the following events?
   A. Nerve action potential
   B. Inhibitory postsynaptic potential (IPSP)
   C. Excitatory postsynaptic potential (EPSP)
   D. Presynaptic inhibition
   E. A and C are correct

225. The outflow from the spinal cord that is the sympathetic nervous system
   A. contains only adrenergic fibers
   B. includes a ganglionic synapse

    C. contains only cholinergic fibers
    D. ceases to function after section of the upper medulla
    E. B and D are correct

226. Alpha waves found in the EEG of a normal person
    A. are associated with restful state
    B. have a frequency of 8 to 12 cps
    C. A and B are correct
    D. are most prominent during intense concentration
    E. all are correct

227. The functions of the basal ganglia include
    A. the inhibition of muscle tone if they are all stimulated
    B. coordinate fine movements of the digits
    C. the globus pallidus is not involved in setting background muscle tone
    D. the caudate nucleus and putamen inhibit gross motor movement
    E. B and D are correct

228. Regarding hippocampal functions
    A. they have reciprocal EEG activity with the cerebral cortex
    B. stimulation and lesions can produce olfactory hallucinations
    C. stimulation while under anesthesia can result in arousal and wakefulness which ceases when the stimulation is turned off
    D. bilateral lesions in humans have suggested memory deficiencies
    E. all are correct

229. Extreme obesity results following lesion of the
    A. supraoptic hypothalamic nucleus
    B. lateral hypothalamic nucleus
    C. ventromedial hypothalamic nucleus
    D. dorsomedial hypothalamic nucleus
    E. none are correct

230. Split brain operations
- **A.** are done routinely on epileptic patients
- **B.** reveal that spatial construction tasks are related to the dominant hemisphere
- **C.** reveal that left hemisphere control of the left hand is extremely refined for the distal musculature
- **D.** are characterized by the contralateral hand being dominant in a task learned by both hands but one hemisphere
- **E.** A and C are correct

231. The pyramidal tract
- **A.** is composed solely of axons from pyramidal cells
- **B.** is a crossed pathway
- **C.** projects solely to the thalamus
- **D.** originates from several areas of the cortex, including area 4, frontal lobe, and the parietal lobe
- **E.** B and D are correct

232. In the cerebellar cortex, which of the following synapses are excitatory?
- **A.** Basket cell on Purkinje cell
- **B.** Climbing fiber on Purkinje cell
- **C.** Descending fiber on Purkinje cell
- **D.** Granule cell on Purkinje cell
- **E.** B and D are correct

233. Cerebral blood flow is altered according to which of the following conditions?
- **A.** Increased physical activity enhances flow
- **B.** Increased mental activity enhances flow
- **C.** Changes with local metabolic needs
- **D.** Increased CO_2 or H^+ concentration causes cerebral vasodilation
- **E.** All of the above

234. Frontal lobe lesions result in
- **A.** signs of complacency, self-satisfaction, and often boastfulness
- **B.** impaired power of judgment of one's situation and narrowing of horizons or goals to the present
- **C.** A and B are correct

D. depression very often

E. all are correct

235. Neuronal inhibition of afferent fibers

    A. can be achieved by presynaptic inhibition

    B. can be achieved by postsynaptic inhibition

    C. A and B are correct

    D. is not a feature of the dorsal column somatosensory system

    E. all are correct

236. Glycine

    A. increases membrane conductance to Cl^- and/or K^+

    B. is blocked by strychnine

    C. hyperpolarizes motoneurons

    D. is present in the terminals of interneuron projections on alpha neurons

    E. all are correct

237. Maximum propagation velocity of the action potential will

    A. be observed in small-diameter fibers

    B. excite skeletal muscle

    C. be observed in unmyelinated fibers

    D. be associated with increased membrane permeability characteristics

    E. A and C are correct

238. The hypothalamus is associated with

    A. food intake

    B. perception

    C. water control

    D. appropriate integration and control of cardiovascular regulation

    E. all of the above

239. The limbic system is involved in

    A. olfaction

    B. rage and fear

    C. A and B are correct

    D. drinking behavior

    E. all are correct

240. Neuronal synapses release ACh that is released from
   A. motoneuron terminals in contact with skeletal muscles
   B. preganglionic nerve terminals to excite postganglionic neurons in contact with the kidney juxtaglomerular cells
   C. A and B are correct
   D. preganglionic nerve terminals to inhibit postganglionic neurons of the autonomic nervous system (ANS)
   E. all are correct

241. Fluid ingestion can be increased by
   A. injections of hypotonic saline into the anterior hypothalamus
   B. psychologic factors
   C. decreased effective osmotic pressure of the plasma
   D. decreased extracellular fluid volume
   E. B and D are correct

242. Sleep deprivation is likely to cause
   A. sluggishness of thought
   B. striking psychologic effects
   C. psychotic episodes
   D. no effect on body function
   E. A, B, and C are correct

243. Dopamine is
   A. related to Parkinsonism as evidenced by the dopamine content of the caudate nucleus and putamen as being about 50% normal
   B. related to prolactin secretion because it is inhibitory and has been used in the treatment of conditions in which there is abnormal milk secretion
   C. involved in pathogenesis of schizophrenia because amphetamines stimulate dopamine secretion producing a psychosis that resembles schizophrenia when administered in large doses
   D. perhaps the prolactin-inhibitory hormone because it has been found in portal hypophyseal blood
   E. all are correct

244. Lesions that produce complete inhibition of fear responses and loss of emotion can often be seen in lesions involving the
   A. sensory cortex
   B. amygdaloid nuclei

    C. olfactory lobes
    D. medulla oblongata
    E. none are correct

245. Recurrent inhibition (inhibitory system) is due to
    A. Renshaw cells which receive recurrent collaterals of motoneurons and inhibit other motoneurons in the vicinity
    B. a major method of lateral inhibition utilized by neurons throughout the CNS
    C. an inhibitory mechanism to sharpen or focus motor output
    D. an inhibitory system of the cerebellum
    E. A, B, and C are correct

246. Hypothermic cooling for cardiac surgery is utilized because
    A. circulation can be stopped for relatively long periods
    B. bleeding is minimal
    C. A and B are correct
    D. blood pressure is normal
    E. all are correct

247. Which of the following is **NOT** a characteristic of spinal cord gray matter organization?
    A. Signals ascend to level of the brain stem and higher
    B. Possesses several million neurons per segment of the spinal cord
    C. Contains interneurons only
    D. Contains interneurons and anterior motor neurons
    E. A and C are correct

248. More than half of the fibers descending and ascending the spinal cord
    A. provide multisegmental reflex pathways
    B. are referred to as propriospinal fibers
    C. include pathways for reflex coordination of simultaneous movement of body parts
    D. are involved in nociception
    E. A, B, and C are correct

249. Which of the following are **NOT** located in the anterior horn of the spinal cord?
   A. Anterior motor neurons
   B. Interneurons
   C. Gamma motor neurons
   D. Alpha motor neurons
   E. None of the above

250. Changes in the basal ganglia result in many clinical syndromes. Which of the following is(are) a syndrome(s) associated with basal ganglia damage or disease?
   A. Athetosis
   B. Chorea
   C. A and B are correct
   D. Dysmetria
   E. All are correct

251. A typical neuron may be characterized accordingly
   A. the dendrites are not electrically excitable and therefore exhibit no action potential
   B. the axon is not electrically excitable and therefore exhibits no action potential
   C. the synaptic afferent fibers are located on the axonic process which is the cell's input zone
   D. it consists of two parts, dendrites and the axon
   E. A and C are correct

252. Which is **NOT** a feature of the central nervous system of mammals?
   A. Spinal cord
   B. Cerebral cortex
   C. Sympathetic post-synaptic neuron
   D. Cerebellum
   E. Brain stem

253. Which of the following may be clinical abnormalities associated with diseases of the cerebellum?
   A. Dysarthria
   B. Ataxia
   C. Dysmetria
   D. Dysdiadochokinesia
   E. All are correct

254. In the perception of pain
  A. the sensation associated with stimuli that leads to tissue damage is referred to as nociception
  B. the relationship between heat transfer to skin and the pain response is curvalinear
  C. the pain stimuli has stimulatory effects on touch and temperature
  D. the neural basis for pain as suggested by the pattern theory is that specific nociceptive transducers exist
  E. A and C are correct

255. The excitatory postsynaptic potential (EPSP) recorded from the cell body of a CNS neuron
  A. lasts only for the duration of the presynaptic action potential
  B. can be spatially summated during repetitive firing of several neurons
  C. is an all-or-none response to a presynaptic impulse
  D. can be temporally summated during repetitive post-synaptic stimulation
  E. B and C are correct

256. In general, opioids
  A. have disinhibitory effects on bulbospinal neurons
  B. mimic the effects of endogenous opioids
  C. A and B are correct
  D. unlike aspirin, act at the level of transduction
  E. all are correct

257. Which of the following is (are) implicated in the initiation of a grand mal attack?
  A. Drugs
  B. Fever
  C. Loud noises
  D. Flashing lights
  E. All are correct

258. Which of the following functions are **NOT** attributable to the level of the spinal cord and/or lower brain?
  A. Walking motions
  B. Reflex control of blood vessels
  C. Equilibrium
  D. Subconscious activities
  E. None of the above

259. Which of the following are **NOT** endogenous opiates of the CNS?
  A. Dynorphin
  B. Beta-endorphin
  C. Haptoglobin
  D. Leu-enkephalin
  E. Beta-lipoprotein

260. Which of the following is **NOT** part of the analgesia system?
  A. Periaqueductal gray matter
  B. Periventricular nuclei of the hypothalamus
  C. Raphe magnus nucleus
  D. Lateral spinothalamic tract
  E. A and C are correct

261. Sensory nerves terminating in the gray matter of the spinal cord
  A. enter the cord through the sensory roots
  B. have facilitory effects
  C. A and B are correct
  D. enter the cord through the corticospinal tract
  E. all are correct

262. Receptive field properties of the striate cortical cells include
  A. orientation selectivity
  B. binocular receptive fields
  C. direction selectivity
  D. motion parallax
  E. A, B, and C are correct

263. Regarding spatial resolution for touch
  A. cutaneous receptive fields are larger where more acute discrimination is needed
  B. cutaneous receptive fields are smaller where more acute discrimination is needed

    C. it is larger for the hand than for the back

    D. is unaffected by afferent inhibition

    E. B and D are correct

264. Deep sleep is or may be

    A. signaled by the appearance of very high-voltage, low-frequency waves on the EEG

    B. associated with a decrease in vegetative functions of the body

    C. the result of synaptic fatigue

    D. the result of a nearly complete lack of input into the cortex from the reticular activating system

    E. all are correct

CNS Physiology

Answers and Discussion

170. (D) Studies of animals (that have survived the removal of the cerebral cortex) have shown conclusively that the capacity to display anger or rage reactions depends on subcortical mechanisms. In studies of both acute and chronic animals, it has been shown that the hypothalamus is necessary for the vigorous expression of rage reactions. (**Ref. 2,** pp. 237–238)

171. (B) A special characteristic of all sensory receptors is that they adapt either partially or completely to their stimuli after a period of time. When a continuous sensory stimulus is applied the receptors respond at a very high impulse rate at first, then progressively less rapidly until finally many of them no longer respond at all. (**Ref. 2,** pp. 107–108)

172. (D) The normal blood flow through brain tissue averages 50–55 mL/100 g of brain per minute. For the entire brain of the average adult, this is approximately 750 mL/min. (**Ref. 2,** pp. 561–564)

173. (D) Dorsal root fibers, upon entering the central nervous system, send branches to many different cells. This divergence makes a single sensory input available to many structures. (**Ref. 2,** pp. 77–78)

174. (D) Since the cerebral cortex is one of the most important areas of the brain for conscious awareness of our surroundings, one can surmise that the ability of specific thalamic areas to excite specific cortical regions might be one of the mechanisms by which a person can direct his attention to specific aspects of his mental environment. (**Ref. 2,** pp. 193–197)

175. (**B**)   The initial reaction during fever is a decreased heat loss because the body does feel cold. Secondarily, there is an increase in heat production. (**Ref. 2,** pp. 231–232)

176. (**D**)   The so-called vomiting center is found in the dorsal part of the lateral reticular formation of the medulla oblongata. (**Ref. 2,** pp. 210–211)

177. (**B**)   The inhibitory synaptic potential involves a selective increase of K^+ or Cl^- but not to Na^+. The synaptic membrane is then less readily depolarized by the action of excitatory presynaptic terminals. (**Ref. 2,** pp. 81–84)

178. (**D**)   During the rising phase of the action potential the major part of the conductance increase is due to sodium. The potassium conductance does not increase appreciably until near the peak of the spike. Thereafter, the sodium conductance decreases rapidly, and a proportionately greater fraction of the total conductance is potassium. (**Ref. 2,** pp. 45–51)

179. (**E**)   Humans tolerate body temperatures of 85°–90°F without permanent ill effects. (**Ref. 2,** p. 232)

180. (**B**)   The somatic sensory area's relationship to the primary motor cortex displays a close functional interdependence of the two areas. It is primarily in the sensory and sensory association areas that one experiences effects of motor movements and records "memories" of the different patterns of motor movements. These are called sensory engrams of the motor movements. (**Ref. 2,** pp. 186–188)

181. (**D**)   The majority of the sympathetic postganglionic endings secrete norepinephrine. (**Ref. 2,** p. 89)

182. (**B**)   There is a preganglionic fiber outflow from each segment of the spinal cord from the first thoracic to the third lumbar level. (**Ref. 2,** pp. 203–205)

183. (A) Some areas anterior to the primary motor cortex that can cause complex coordinate movements, such as speech, eye movements, and head movements, are referred to as the premotor cortex. **(Ref. 2,** p. 187)

184. (C) The motor cortex can be considered as four separate motor areas: the primary motor, supplementary motor, somatic sensorimotor I, and somatic sensorimotor Il. **(Ref. 2,** pp. 186–188)

185. (E) When the rectal temperature is over 41° C (106° F) for prolonged periods, some permanent brain damage results. **(Ref. 2,** pp. 231–232)

186. (B) The number of vesicles released with each action potential is greatly reduced when the quantity of calcium ions in the extracellular fluid is diminished. It has been suggested that the spread of the action potential over the membrane of the knob causes small amounts of calcium ions to leak into the knob. The calcium ions then supposedly attract the transmitter vesicles to the membrane and simultaneously cause one or more of them to rupture, thus allowing spillage of their contents into the synaptic cleft. **(Ref. 2,** pp. 76–78)

187. (E) By far the majority of the reticular formation is excitatory. Diffuse stimulation of facilitory areas causes a general increase in muscle tone throughout the body or in localized areas. In the normal animal, inhibitory signals are continually available from the basal ganglia, cerebellum, and the cerebral cortex to keep the facilitory system from becoming overactive. **(Ref. 2,** pp. 174–175)

188. (C) EEG patterns become rapid, of low voltage, and irregular, and these resemble the EEGs seen in alert humans. The threshold for arousal by sensory stimuli is elevated. This condition is called paradoxical sleep. **(Ref. 2,** pp. 176–177)

189. (A) The inhibitory influences of the deep cerebellar nuclei arise entirely from the Purkinje cells in the cortex of the cerebellum. All of the efferent tracts from the cerebellum arise in the deep nuclei; none arise from the cerebellar cortex. **(Ref. 2,** pp. 197–202)

190. (B) A pair of electrodes placed on the surface of an uninjured nerve will record a zero potential followed by a diphasic compound action potential. (**Ref. 2,** pp. 46–50)

191. (B) The EPSP is a local depolarization of the postjunctional membrane caused by a transient increase in the ionic permeability of this membrane. The action of ACh on the postjunctional membrane is to increase its permeability to all species of ions. (**Ref. 2,** pp. 79–80)

192. (A) Since the pump requires energy for operation, this process of "recharging" the nerve fiber is an active metabolic one, utilizing energy from the ATP energy "currency" system of the cell. (**Ref. 2,** p. 51)

193. (C) The cerebellum receives an extensive afferent pathway by the corticocerebellar pathway, which originates mainly in the motor cortex (but to a lesser extent in the sensory cortex as well). It then passes by way of the pontile nuclei and pontocerebellar tracts directly to the cortex of the cerebellum. (**Ref. 2,** pp. 197–202)

194. (A) GABA appears to have a true hyperpolarization at the lateral vestibular nucleus and cerebral and cerebellar cortices, except that its action is resistant to strychnine. In the crustacean peripheral inhibitory motor fibers, GABA is already convincingly identified as the inhibitory transmitter. (**Ref. 2,** p. 96)

195. (E) Certain alpha functions are excitatory, while others are inhibitory. Therefore, alpha and beta receptors are not associated with excitation or inhibition, but simply with the affinity of the hormones for the receptors in a given organ. (**Ref. 2,** p. 91)

196. (E) The medullary center is under the influence of chemical changes in the blood, blood pressure alterations, afferent impulses from the viscera, and higher control centers. White blood cell concentration in the blood has no direct effect upon the centers. (**Ref. 2,** pp. 546–552)

197. (A) When excited, the eating centers that are associated with hunger are the perifornical and lateral nucleus of the hypothalamus. Damage to these areas causes the animal to lose desire for food. A center that reduces the desire for food is called the satiety center. These hypothalamic nuclei may be served by glucose receptors. (**Ref. 2,** pp. 215–217)

198. **(C)** Presynaptic inhibition is caused by the presence of inhibitory knobs lying directly on the terminal fibrils and excitatory knobs themselves. They secrete a transmitter substance that partially depolarizes the terminal fibrils and the excitatory synaptic knobs. Consequently, the voltage of the action potential that occurs at the membrane of the excitatory knob is depressed, and this greatly reduces the amount of excitatory transmitter released at the knob. (**Ref. 2,** pp. 81–84)

199. **(A)** At the cathode, the potential outside the membrane is negative with respect to that on the inside. Current flows outward through the anode. Cathodal current decreases, while an anodal current actually increases resistance to excitation. The all-or-none principle of excitation is based on the finding that electrical stimulation has a strength limit above which a full action potential results with propogation. (**Ref. 2,** pp. 47–48)

200. **(E)** With time, the depression of segmental reflexes disappears. Usually, the first reflexes to return after a period of spinal shock are the flexion reflexes mediated by polysynaptic pathways. (**Ref. 2,** pp. 189–191)

201. **(B)** One type of focal epilepsy is the so-called psychomotor seizure, which may cause (1) a short period of amnesia; (2) an attack of abnormal rage; (3) sudden anxiety, discomfort, or fear; (4) a moment of incoherent speech or mumbling of some trite phrase; or (5) a motor act to attack someone, to rub the face with the hand, or so forth. (**Ref. 2,** pp. 182–183)

202. **(E)** Examination of a patient who has sustained unilateral anterolateral cordotomy reveals several sensory changes. First, contralateral loss of pain and temperature sensation. Motor components would reflect a typical upper motoneuron lesion set of symptoms. (**Ref. 2,** pp. 122–132)

203. **(E)** The thalamic syndrome involves emotional changes, various degrees of anesthesia, and motor symptoms such as ataxia. There is

also a permanent loss or severe impairment of light touch and position as well as a delay in the recognition of superficial stimuli. Sexual functions are not altered in thalamic lesions. (**Ref. 2,** pp. 174–183)

204. (**B**)   The usual course is for petit mal attacks to appear in late childhood and then to disappear entirely by the age of 30. Petit mal will often become grand mal, since both originate in the same locus. (**Ref. 2,** pp. 182–183)

205. (**E**)   Sleep or sleep-like behavior can be produced by stimulation of the thalamic intralaminar nuclei, the preoptic and supraoptic areas, and the caudate. The existence of a wakefulness center is questionable. The ventral posterolateral nucleus of the thalamus has no relationship to sleep. (**Ref. 2,** pp. 178–182)

206. (**E**)   Some of the hypothalamic lesion syndromes include the hyperthermic syndrome, the diabetes insipidus and emaciation syndrome, the adiposogenital dystrophy syndrome, the syndrome characterized by somnolence and disorder of temperature regulation, and finally diencephalic or autonomic epilepsy. In no case will psychosis be found in hypothalamic lesions. (**Ref. 2,** pp. 367–378)

207. (**E**)   The common denominator of most cerebellar signs is inappropriate rate, range, force, and direction of movement. Lack of reflexes (areflexia) is not a cerebellar symptom. (**Ref. 2,** pp. 197–202)

208. (**A**)   Stimulation of the nervous system results in increased, copious sweating, whereas with atropine there is a decreased secretion of sweat glands. Parasympathetic stimulation does not influence ventricular inotropicity. (**Ref. 2,** pp. 203–209)

209. (**C**)   Release of neurotransmitter into the synaptic cleft may result in either of two responses: inhibition or excitation of the postsynaptic membrane. An increase in intraneuronal voltage from the normal resting potential (i.e., resting membrane potential becomes more negative) caused by a neurotransmitter, indicates a hyperpolarized state. This is called inhibitory postsynaptic potential (IPSP). Because of the structural and integrative properties of neurons, synaptic inputs (both EPSPs and IPSPs) can occur by either spatial or temporal summation. In either case there is a change in the concentration of calcium ions, which mediates the release of neurotransmitter in the synaptic cleft. (**Ref. 2,** pp. 79–81)

210. **(A)** The electrical events that occur in the cortex after stimulation of a sense organ can be monitored with an exploring electrode connected to the reference electrode. The first positive–negative wave sequence is the primary evoked potential; the second is the diffuse secondary response. (**Ref. 2,** pp. 175–176)

211. **(B)** Care should be taken to avoid damaging the nuclei when surgical removal of parts of the cerebellum is necessary. Compensation for the effects of cortical lesions occurs, but compensation for the effects of lesions of the cerebellar nuclei does not occur. (**Ref. 2,** pp. 197–202)

212. **(E)** True active hypersomnia with accompanying slow-wave sleep and paradoxical sleep is due to increased release of serotonin. (**Ref. 2,** pp. 178–183)

213. **(C)** Usually the first reflexes to return after a period of spinal shock are the flexion reflexes mediated by polysynaptic pathways. (**Ref. 2,** pp. 189–191)

214. **(B)** Sweat glands are innervated by sympathetic cholinergic postganglionic fibers. (**Ref. 2,** p. 207)

215. **(A)** The peripheral neuropathy associated with alcoholism and deficiency of vitamin B_1 selects small fibers and produces a modality dissociation.

216. **(E)** Neuroglia are almost exclusively permeable to potassium ions. The potential gradient is established between depolarized glia, where extracellular potassium is high, and adjacent glia cells. The resulting current flow through bridges of low resistance tend to remove potassium from clefts where the concentration of this ion is high. This method of buffering the extracellular potassium concentration is one possible role of the glia scar formation. These sites are often areas of epileptic activity. (**Ref. 2,** pp. 182–183)

217. **(C)** Parasympathetic stimulation causes myosis and increases glandular secretion and HCl secretion by the stomach. (**Ref. 2,** pp. 203–209)

218. **(B)** After destruction of the amygdaloid nucleus and lumbar system, the normal fear reaction is often absent. **(Ref. 2, p. 237)**

219. **(A)** Purkinje cells are always inhibitory influences on the tonically active neurons of the cerebellar nuclei. **(Ref. 2, pp. 199–200)**

220. **(E)** Because a synapse represents a physical "gap" between presynaptic and postsynaptic membranes, there is a time barrier which is a function of that distance. The time required for a neurotransmitter to traverse this distance is referred to as synaptic delay. Unlike axonal transmission of action potentials, which can travel in both directions along its length, synaptic transmission is in one direction, due to the presynaptic and postsynaptic arrangement of secretory vesicle and receptors, respectively. Axonal potentials exhibit the all-or-none principle while synapses summate algebraically, adding excitatory while subtracting inhibitory potentials. **(Ref. 2, pp. 84–101)**

221. **(C)** When the sodium channels open and these ions pour through the membrane, the positive charges of the sodium ions neutralize the normal electronegativity inside the fiber and also create an excess of positive charges. Hence, the membrane potential inside the fibers is positive and is called the reversal potential at about the time K^+ permeability increases and repolarization is initiated. **(Ref. 2, pp. 46–51)**

222. **(B)** Paradoxical sleep is usually associated with active dreaming. **(Ref. 2, pp. 178–183)**

223. **(C)** Drugs that mimic the action of norepinephrine on sympathetic effector organs have shown that there are at least two different types of adrenergic receptors. **(Ref. 2, pp. 91, 206–207)**

224. **(A)** Under the same resting conditions a nerve action potential will always have the same amplitude. **(Ref. 2, p. 47)**

225. **(B)** A sympathetic path always contains a preganglionic and postganglionic neuron. **(Ref. 2, pp. 204, 213–214)**

226. **(C)** Alpha waves are seen most often in a resting but awake person. They occur 8 to 12 times per second. **(Ref. 2, pp. 176–177)**

227. (A) Fine control of the digits is dependent on the function of the primary motor cortex. (**Ref. 2,** pp. 185–188)

228. (E) Investigators who have studied behavioral effects in the monkey consequent to bilateral destruction of the amygdaloid nuclei, uncus, or hippocampi have found that the animals were tame, fearless, and asocial for 4 to 5 months. (**Ref. 2,** pp. 237–239)

229. (C) Destruction or anesthetization of the ventromedial nuclei leads to acceleration of self-stimulation and feeding. (**Ref. 2,** pp. 215–216)

230. (D) Split brain operations on humans have revealed that in a task learned by a single hemisphere, but where both hands are part of the learned task, the contralateral hand will be dominant. (**Ref. 2,** p. 245)

231. (E) The pyramidal tract is a crossed pathway with a diffuse origin. (**Ref. 2,** p. 185)

232. (E) Climbing fibers and granule cells are excitatory to the Purkinje cell in the cerebellar cortex. (**Ref. 2,** pp. 199–200)

233. (E) Adjustment of cerebral blood flow in accordance with local requirements of cerebral metabolism is well documented. Increases in carbon dioxide or hydrogen ion concentration will dilate cerebral arterioles and thereby increase flow. (**Ref. 2,** pp. 561–565)

234. (C) Many patients exhibit tactlessness, extroversion, euphoria, and noticeable lability of emotions with a tendency to outbursts. (**Ref. 2,** pp. 233–253)

235. (C) Afferent inhibition is a prominent feature of the dorsal column somatosensory system. It can be achieved by presynaptic and postsynaptic inhibition. A volley of impulses in dorsal root afferents leaves in its wake an enduring depolarization of the intraspinal segments of both the active and the adjacent fibers. (**Ref. 2,** pp. 81–84)

236. (E) Certain characteristics of physiologic inhibitory transmission, including true hyperpolarization and increased membrane conductance to Cl^- or K^+, that are antagonized by strychnine and related compounds have been produced by glycine. Glycine is an inhibitory transmitter. (**Ref. 2,** pp. 96–97)

237. (**B**) The velocity of conduction in nerve fibers varies from as little as 0.5 m/s in very small unmyelinated fibers up to as high as 130 m/s in very large myelinated fibers. The velocity increases approximately with the fiber diameter in myelinated nerve fibers and approximately with the square root of fiber diameter in unmyelinated fibers. The excitation of nodes permits the saltatory conduction and muscle excitation. (**Ref. 2,** pp. 48–53)

238. (**E**) The hypothalamus is of importance to the perception of thirst and the control of water intake. It is also involved in the regulation of body water loss, partially via the kidney. (**Ref. 2,** pp. 211–224)

239. (**C**) Stimulation and ablation experiments indicate that in addition to its role in olfaction, the limbic system is concerned with feeding behavior. Along with the hypothalamus, it is also concerned with sexual behavior and the emotions of rage, fear, and motivation. (**Ref. 2,** pp. 233–239)

240. (**C**) (**Ref. 2,** pp. 76–77)

241. (**B**) Drinking can be increased by increased effective osmotic pressure of the plasma, by decreases in ECF volume, and by psychologic and other factors. Injections of hypertonic saline into the anterior hypothalamus causes drinking in conscious animals. (**Ref. 2,** pp. 221–223)

242. (**E**) Prolonged wakefulness is often associated with progressive malfunction of the mind and behavioral activities of the nervous system. A person can become irritable or even psychotic following forced wakefulness for prolonged periods of time. (**Ref. 2,** pp. 178–183)

243. (**E**) The physiologic role of dopamine is related to Parkinsonism because dopamine content of the caudate nucleus and putamen is about 50% normal. It is related to prolactin secretion because it is inhibitory and has been used in the treatment of conditions in which there is abnormal milk secretion. Pathogenesis of schizophrenia has been postulated because amphetamines, which stimulate dopamine secretion, produce a psychosis that resembles schizophrenia when administered in large doses. It may actually be the prolactin-inhibitory hormone because it has been found in portal hypophyseal blood. It is not related to the opiate receptors or pain. (**Ref. 2,** pp. 91, 196–197)

244. **(B)** The fear reaction and its autonomic and endocrine manifestations are absent in situations in which they would normally be evoked when the amygdala is destroyed. (**Ref. 2,** p. 237)

245. **(E)** Small interneurons, called Renshaw cells, lie in close association with motoneurons. Motoneuron axon collaterals pass to Renshaw cells, which in turn transmit inhibitory signals to nearby motoneurons. Both sensory and motor systems utilize lateral inhibition to sharpen and focus their signals. (**Ref. 2,** pp. 179–180)

246. **(C)** When the skin or blood is cooled enough to lower the body temperature in humans, metabolic and physiologic processes slow down. Respiration and heart rates are very slow, blood pressure is low, bleeding is minimal, and consciousness is lost. These conditions are excellent for surgery. (**Ref. 2,** p. 232)

247. **(C)** In each segment of the spinal cord there are several million neurons in its gray matter. Each segment of the anterior horn of gray matter contains several thousand anterior motor neurons, 50% to 100% larger than most others. Included are interneurons. The neurons of gray matter may travel to higher levels in the cord itself, to the brain stem, or even to the level of the cerebral cortex. (**Ref. 2,** pp. 203–204)

248. **(E)** The multiple segmental interconnecting fibers of the spinal cord are referred to as the propriospinal fibers and comprise more than half of the fibers of the spinal cord. Both ascending and descending, they include reflexes for coordinated control of the simultaneous movement of fore and hind limbs. (**Ref. 2,** pp. 203–204)

249. **(E)** All of the neurons listed are located in all areas of the gray matter, including the anterior horn. (**Ref. 2,** pp. 203–204)

250. **(C)** Chorea is characterized by random uncontrolled "flicking" movements. Athetosis is slow "worm-like" writhing movements of the neck, face, and hands. Dysmetria is a condition associated with diseases of the cerebellum. (**Ref. 2,** pp. 196–197)

251. **(A)** The neuron has three distinct regions: dendritic processes, soma, and axon. The dendrites represent the input zone and the axon represents the cells sole means of output. The soma and dendrites are not electrically excitable in that they do not display voltage-dependent conductance and therefore do not show an action potential. On the other hand the axon displays all these features. (**Ref. 2,** pp. 43–45)

252. **(C)** Sympathetic post-synaptic neurons are part of the peripheral nervous system. (**Ref. 2,** pp. 203–205)

253. **(E)** All listed. (**Ref. 2,** pp. 197–202)

254. **(A)** There are theories, including the pattern theory and gate control theories, for the pain response. The most widely accepted is the specific theory, which suggests that there are specific nociceptive transducers that are actually responsible for the pain response. However, the perception of pain may include aspects of all three theories. It is also known that pain can have inhibitory effects on touch and temperature perception. (**Ref. 2,** pp. 126–131)

255. **(B)** When an afferent volley to the cerebral cortex is either purely excitatory or purely inhibitory for a cell under stimulation, that cell responds with EPSPs that are depolarizing or hyperpolarizing. These can summate spatially and/or temporally but it is not an all or none response. (**Ref. 2,** pp. 79–80)

256. **(C)** Opioids like morphine act centrally and mimic the endogenous opioids. Generally, they have inhibitory effects on neurons. However, the bulbospinal neurons block nociception when activated. It is believed that opioids activate the bulbospinal neurons by disinhibition. Aspirin, a true analgesic, works at the level of transduction. (**Ref. 2,** pp. 97–98)

257. **(E)** All the factors listed can initiate a grand mal attack in those individuals so predisposed. However, in individuals not predisposed genetically, traumatic lesions in almost any part of the brain can cause excess excitability in local brain areas. These may trans-

mit signal into the reticular activating system eliciting a grand mal attack. (**Ref. 2,** pp. 182–183)

258. **(E)** Functions associated with the level of the spinal cord include withdrawal reflexes and support against gravity but equilibrium and subconscious activities are functions of the lower brain level: medulla, cerebellum, and basal ganglia. (**Ref. 2,** pp. 184–191)

259. **(C)** All listed but haptoglobin. (**Ref. 2,** pp. 97–98)

260. **(D)** The lateral spinothalamic tract is part of the anterolateral system for transmission of sensory signals that do not require discrimination of intensity or discrete localization. (**Ref. 2,** p. 130)

261. **(C)** The sensory signal enters the spinal cord through the sensory roots. Their effects include local segmental and excitatory responses, facilitory effects, and reflexes. (**Ref. 2,** pp. 122–123)

262. **(E)** Motion parallax is a phenomenon associated with monocular cues of depth, specifically, the retinal image of objects moving at different rates and at different distances. (**Ref. 2,** pp. 193–194)

263. **(B)** Spatial resolution is defined as the minimal separation for two stimuli to be distinguished as one. Where tactile acuity is more important, receptive fields are smaller, such as for the hand, and where tactile acuity is not so important, receptive fields are larger, as for the body trunk. Unlike primary cutaneous afferent fibers, neurons of the dorsal column, somatosensory cortex, and ventral posterolateral nuclei possess lateral inhibition; stimuli in one area inhibits excitation in surrounding zonal regions. (**Ref. 2,** pp. 122–125)

264. **(E)** Deep sleep is characterized by high-voltage delta waves occurring at a rate of 1 to 2 per second. It is dreamless, associated with a decrease in both peripheral vascular tone and most of the other vegetative functions of the body as well. It may be due to synaptic decay and is probably due to a nearly complete lack of input by which a person can direct his attention to specific aspects of his mental environment. (**Ref. 2,** pp. 178–182)

4

Respiratory Physiology

MULTIPLE CHOICE

DIRECTIONS (Questions 265–323): Each of the questions or incomplete statements below is followed by five suggested answers or completions. Select the **one** that is **best** in each case.

265. A patient has a long-standing problem of diabetes mellitus (insulin deficiency) which you have been able to stabilize with daily insulin therapy. Suddenly this patient goes into a condition of severe acidosis and is brought into the hospital. You should **EXPECT** which of the following laboratory findings?

   A. A decrease in plasma pH, an increase in plasma HCO_3^-, and an acidic urine
   B. A decrease in plasma HCO_3^-, an increase in plasma pH, and an acid urine
   C. A urine that is acidic, a decrease in plasma HCO_3^-, and a decrease in plasma pH
   D. A urine that is alkaline, a decrease in plasma HCO_3^-, and a decrease in plasma pH
   E. Depressed respiration

266. In severe exercise the oxygen debt is
- **A.** surplus O_2 borrowed from the inspiratory reserve during exercise
- **B.** the average O_2 used less the resting O_2 for a similar time; required for anaerobic processes
- **C.** O_2 used above resting levels borrowed to provide the increased aerobic oxidations
- **D.** O_2 used after exercise above resting level and representing in part the anaerobic contribution in work
- **E.** decreased

267. Which of the following sets of values is indicative of compensated metabolic alkalosis?
- **A.** $HCO_3^- = 20$ mEq/L, $pCO_2 = 25$ mm Hg, pH = 7.5
- **B.** $HCO_3^- = 42$ mEq/L, $pCO_2 = 45$ mm Hg, pH = 7.5
- **C.** $HCO_3^- = 17$ mEq/L, $pCO_2 = 30$ mm Hg, pH = 7.3
- **D.** $HCO_3^- = 34$ mEq/L, $pCO_2 = 10$ mm Hg, pH = 7.7
- **E.** $HCO_3^- = 17$ mEq/L, $pCO_2 = 19$ mm Hg, pH = 7.9

268. You are examining a patient who has an arterial pCO_2 of 40 mm Hg. During a test period the pCO_2 of expired gas is found to be 20 mm Hg and a respiratory minute volume of 8 L is noted. From these data the
- **A.** alveolar ventilation is 8 L/min
- **B.** alveolar ventilation is 40 L/min
- **C.** alveolar ventilation is 4 L/min
- **D.** tidal volume is 8 L
- **E.** test should be stopped before potentially fatal cardiac arrhythmias occur

269. Respiratory alkalosis is characterized by
- **A.** low pH concentration
- **B.** fall in pCO_2
- **C.** excess pulmonary ventilation
- **D.** protein synthesis increases
- **E.** reduced HCO_3^-/pCO_2 rate

270. Dynamic collapse of airways occurs
- **A.** during vigorous inspiration
- **B.** mostly in the respiratory bronchioles where walls are thin
- **C.** in major bronchi during violent expiration because these airways have lower internal pressures than do smaller airways further upstream (nearer the alveoli)

D. only in unusual disease conditions
E. during normal quiet expiration

271. The primary stimulus of respiration is a
    A. two-fold increase in the pCO_2 of inspired air
    B. two-fold increase in the pO_2 of inspired air
    C. 50% decrease in the pCO_2 of inspired air
    D. 50% increase in the pO_2 of inspired air
    E. 50% decrease in pCO_2

272. The periodic nature of normal respiration is fundamentally caused by
    A. intermittent bursts of activity from cells in the pontine "apneustic center"
    B. feedback loops involving the peripheral chemoceptors
    C. coupled oscillatory behavior of inspiratory and expiratory cells in the medulla
    D. "pneumotaxic center"
    E. conscious control from areas of the motor cortex

273. The limitation of the pulmonary diffusion process
    A. is no movement of the molecules through the alveolar gas phase
    B. involves CO_2 equilibrium across the alveolar membrane
    C. prevents normal individuals from ever reaching alveolar-capillary pO_2 equilibrium
    D. is determined by reaction kinetics of the O_2 hemoglobin association and by O_2 solubility
    E. is largely determined by the diffusion capacity of the alveolar capillary membrane and capillary plasma

274. You are presented with a patient that you suspect has a compensated metabolic acidosis. Which of the following sets of lab data would confirm your suspicion?
    A. $HCO_3^- = 17$ mEq/L, $pCO_2 = 19$ mm Hg, pH = 7.9
    B. $HCO_3^- = 34$ mEq/L, $pCO_2 = 10$ mm Hg, pH = 7.7
    C. $HCO_3^- = 17$ mEq/L, $pCO_2 = 30$ mm Hg, pH = 7.3
    D. $HCO_3^- = 24$ mEq/L, $pCO_2 = 45$ mm Hg, pH = 7.5
    E. $HCO_3^- = 20$ mEq/L, $pCO_2 = 25$ mm Hg, pH = 7.5

275. Breathing CO_2 for prolonged periods results in
  A. only alveolar pCO_2 rises
  B. only tissue pCO_2 decreases
  C. alveolar ventilation decreases
  D. both alveolar and tissue pCO_2 increase
  E. liver cirrhosis

276. In contrast to the systemic circulation, the pulmonary circulation is characterized by
  A. low mean pressure
  B. high resistance
  C. relative small pulse pressure
  D. large volume flow per minute
  E. absence of sympathetic control

277. The total quantity of air that can be expelled from the lungs following a maximal inspiration is known as the
  A. vital capacity
  B. tidal volume
  C. expiratory reserve volume
  D. functional residual capacity
  E. total capacity

278. Which of the following is true regarding respiration?
  A. Influenced by centers located in the medulla
  B. Controlled by centers located in the cerebellum
  C. At the end of inspiration the pressure in the alveolar space within the lungs is atmospheric
  D. At the end of expiration the pressure in the alveolar space within the lungs is subatmospheric
  E. A and C are correct

279. CO_2 is carried by the blood in the following ways **EXCEPT**
  A. in physical solution with the plasma
  B. bound to non-heme protein
  C. in the form of bicarbonate
  D. in combination with hemoglobin
  E. B and D are correct

280. Which is **NOT** a feature influencing O_2 delivery and CO_2 removal from the body?
  A. Interaction among sensory receptors located in the lungs
  B. Interaction among sensory receptors located in the arteries
  C. Changes in intrathoracic pressure during the breathing cycle
  D. The churning action of gas within the lung created by contractions of the heart
  E. None of the above

281. During contraction of the diaphragm
  A. the intra-abdominal pressure becomes negative
  B. the diaphragm flattens
  C. the vertical dimensions of the thoracic cage decrease
  D. the lateral dimensions of the thoracic cage decrease
  E. B and D are correct

282. The diaphragm
  A. accounts for half the inspired air during inspiration
  B. accounts for less than one third of the inspired air during anesthesia
  C. is supplied by the vagus nerve
  D. is over two-thirds made up of slow-twitch fibers which resist fatigue
  E. B and D are correct

283. To determine the cost of breathing
  A. oxygen consumption is measured at rest and at increased ventilation
  B. oxygen consumption is measured before and after exercise
  C. normally it is 25% of the total O_2 consumed by the body
  D. oxygen consumption is decreased as the elasticity of the chest bellows increases
  E. A and C are correct

284. Functional residual capacity is
  A. the volume of air exhaled during exhalation
  B. the amount of air left in the lungs at the end of normal, resting expiration
  C. the volume of air inhaled during inspiration
  D. the maximal amount of air that can be exhaled after quiet expiration
  E. none of the above

285. The volume of air contained in the lungs
 A. after maximal expiration is the residual volume
 B. after maximal inspiration is termed expiratory reserve volume (ERV)
 C. after maximal inspiration from functional residual capacity is inspiratory capacity (IC)
 D. A and C are correct
 E. all are correct

286. Which of the following is true regarding the elastic properties of the lung?
 A. Collagen and elastin are responsible for the resilience of the lung
 B. In diseases that decrease distensibility, the elastic recoil exceeds that of the normal lung
 C. A and B are correct
 D. Emphysema decreases the distensibility of the lung
 E. All are correct

287. The elastic recoil of the chest wall
 A. is directed inward at end-inspiration
 B. is directed outward at functional residual capacity
 C. is opposed by the recoil of the lungs
 D. is approximately 70% of lung capacity at equilibrium
 E. all are correct

288. Fluid flow through the circulatory system is in many respects similar to fluid flow through a tube, in that
 A. flow rate is faster near the center of flow
 B. it is directly proportional to the square of the diameter of the tube
 C. it is always characterized by laminar flow
 D. flow rate is directly proportional to length of the tube
 E. A and C are correct

289. Which of the following is (are) true regarding air and water flow through a tube?
 A. Air molecules are free to collide more randomly and therefore form eddies much more readily
 B. Air flow rate is proportional to the square root of the driving pressure

C. A and B are correct
D. Air flow rate is independent of density
E. All are correct

290. Which of the following is **TRUE** regarding distribution of airway resistance in respiration?
    A. Total cross-sectional area increases with each successive branching
    B. Airway resistance decreases with each successive branching
    C. Greater during nose breathing than mouth breathing
    D. Greater in the subsegmental regions than in upper trachea or bronchial tree
    E. A and C are correct

291. At the beginning of forced expiration
    A. intrathoracic airways widen
    B. transmural airway pressure decreases
    C. lung elastic recoil increases
    D. airway resistance decreases
    E. B and D are correct

292. During a maximal inspiratory event
    A. force generation of the muscles of inspiration increases
    B. the transmural pressure remains low
    C. the pleural pressure is subatmospheric
    D. flow rate remains high, but only over a narrow range of lung volumes
    E. all are correct

293. Most of the venous CO_2 is in the form of
    A. carbamino compounds
    B. dissolved CO_2
    C. bicarbonate
    D. carbonic acid
    E. A and C are correct

294. The oxygen dissociation curve is shifted to the right by
    A. decreased pCO_2
    B. increased 2,3-DPG (2,3-diphosphoglycerate)
    C. decreased blood temperature
    D. increased pH
    E. B and D are correct

295. Alveolar space pressure is
   A. less than atmospheric pressure during expiration as a consequence of lung compliance
   B. independent of airflow direction and airway dimensions
   C. subatmospheric at the end of inspiration
   D. dependent upon airway dimensions and direction of airflow
   E. B and D are correct

296. Severe hypoventilation will result from
   A. an abnormally low alveolar pCO_2
   B. direct stimulation of medullary chemoreceptors by hypoxia
   C. A and B are correct
   D. cyanosis and alkalosis of systemic arterial blood
   E. all are correct

297. Hyperpnea resulting from moderate exercise may be due to
   A. increased body temperature
   B. joint movement
   C. serum pH increase
   D. decrease in serum pCO_2
   E. A and C are correct

298. The diffusion of oxygen across the alveolar membrane is much less than that of CO_2 because
   A. the alveolar area available for O_2 diffusion is larger
   B. CO_2 is more soluble in H_2O (than is O_2), which enables it to pass the membrane easier
   C. CO_2 is actively transferred
   D. the molecular weight of O_2 is greater than CO_2
   E. B and D are correct

299. Loss of or decreased vagal activity results in a(n)
   A. loss of some sensory input to the respiratory centers
   B. a regular breathing pattern
   C. increased rate of respiration
   D. decreased depth of respiration
   E. all are correct

300. A patient presents with severe prolonged vomiting from deep inside the gastrointestinal tract. The most likely consequence(s) is (are)
  - **A.** increase in rate and depth of respiration
  - **B.** metabolic acidosis
  - **C.** decrease in plasma pH
  - **D.** increase in plasma bicarbonate
  - **E.** all are correct

301. Hemoglobin is particularly well suited to carry oxygen in the blood. Its advantages in the human include
  - **A.** the leftward shift in affinity that results from acid conditions
  - **B.** a greater affinity for O_2 than for carbon monoxide
  - **C.** an easily reversible binding with O_2
  - **D.** the ability to give up most of its oxygen at pO_2 between 5 and 20 mm Hg
  - **E.** A and C are correct

302. Oxygen release from hemoglobin is caused and enhanced by
  - **A.** low temperature in the tissues
  - **B.** high pCO_2 in the tissues
  - **C.** high pH in the tissues
  - **D.** low pO_2 in the tissues
  - **E.** B and D are correct

303. Carbon monoxide
  - **A.** loosely combines with CO_2 in the plasma
  - **B.** interferes with CO_2 transport
  - **C.** has a lesser affinity to combine with hemoglobin than does oxygen
  - **D.** interferes with O_2 transport
  - **E.** A and C are correct

304. Hering-Breuer reflexes result in
  - **A.** inhibition of inspiration when the lungs are inflated
  - **B.** excitation of inspiration when the lungs are inflated
  - **C.** excitation of inspiration when the lungs are deflated
  - **D.** inhibition of inspiration when the lungs are deflated
  - **E.** A and C are correct

305. The total oxygen in the blood will
  A. be most closely related to the pO_2 of the blood
  B. be most closely related to the hemoglobin content
  C. not be reduced in hypoxia
  D. be increased in anemia
  E. none are correct

306. The compliance of a lung that changes in volume 1 L when the intrapleural pressure is lowered by 5 cm of H_2O would be
  A. calculated by dividing $\Delta P/\Delta V$
  B. calculated by multiplying $\Delta V \times \Delta P$
  C. .20 L/cm of H_2O
  D. 5.0 L/cm of H_2O
  E. A and C are correct

307. Perfusion without ventilation
  A. acts like an increased partial pressure of oxygen in the alveoli
  B. acts like an arteriovenous shunt
  C. acts like an increase in dead space
  D. leads to an increase in oxygen in the alveoli involved
  E. B and D are correct

308. The ventilation perfusion ratio (V/Q)
  A. is determined by dividing the total alveolar ventilation by the cardiac output
  B. is determined by dividing cardiac output by alveolar ventilation
  C. in a patient with cardiac output of 12 L/min and alveolar ventilation of 2 L/min would be equal to 6
  D. is a constant for a given individual
  E. A and C are correct

309. The pontine respiratory center has
  A. its effects through a cortical-medullary reflex arc
  B. an area that will cause prolonged expiration if stimulated
  C. an area that is primarily active in controlling the rate of respiration
  D. afferents directly to motoneurons necessary for respiration
  E. A and C are correct

310. When a patient has an extremely low arterial pO_2
   A. normal respiration cannot occur
   B. the CNS will be directly stimulated
   C. the aortic body is most responsible for sensing the condition
   D. the presentation of 100% O_2 can be catastrophic
   E. B and D are correct

311. Chemoreceptor drive constitutes an important compensatory mechanism in
   A. anemia
   B. methemoglobinemia
   C. carbon monoxide poisoning
   D. emphysema
   E. B and D are correct

312. The work of breathing is made up in part by work
   A. required to overcome inertia of tissues
   B. required to stretch elastic elements in the chest
   C. necessary to overcome airway resistance
   D. necessary to hold the bronchi open
   E. A, B, and C are correct

313. Dyspnea is
   A. the sensation of inadequate or distressful breathing
   B. normal resting breathing
   C. increased breath rate and depth
   D. A and C are correct
   E. all are correct

314. In Figure 12 the greatest change in volume during expiration and inspiration would occur at site(s)
   A. A, B, and C
   B. B and D
   C. C and E
   D. C and D
   E. D only

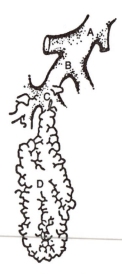

Figure 12

315. In Figure 13,
   A. curve Y is at a higher pH than curve X
   B. curve X is at a higher pH than curve Y
   C. the somewhat S-shaped curves are due to the effect of CO_2 on hemoglobin
   D. the somewhat S-shaped curves are due to a changing affinity of oxygen by hemoglobin at increasing 2,3-DPG (2,3-diphosphoglycerate) concentration
   E. B and D are correct

316. In Figure 13 a shift from curve Y to curve Z would occur if peripheral tissues developed a higher
   A. temperature
   B. 2,3-DPG (2,3-diphosphoglycerate)
   C. A and B are correct
   D. myoglobin content
   E. all are correct

317. The diaphragm
   A. decreases the volume of the thoracic space when it contracts
   B. decreases intrathoracic pressure when it contracts
   C. is innervated by the vagus nerve
   D. increases intrathoracic pressure when it contracts
   E. B and D are correct

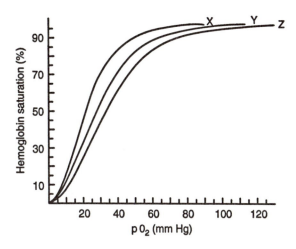

Figure 13

318. Lung surfactant
   A. decreases the likelihood of alveolar collapse during expiration
   B. facilitates O_2 diffusion through alveolar membranes
   C. facilitates CO_2 diffusion through alveolar membranes
   D. increases surface tension of the alveolar membrane
   E. A and C are correct

319. Within the lungs the molecules of any gas
   A. that develop a pressure will have a pressure whose magnitude is determined by the number of molecules present
   B. collide with other molecules that rebound, which results in a "pressure" development
   C. are in continuous motion
   D. do not move randomly nor can they develop a pressure
   E. A, B, and C are correct

320. There are several factors controlling adult human respiration on a moment-to-moment basis. Those which are of importance include
   A. pulmonary stretch reflexes
   B. systemic arterial pCO_2 on carotid and aortic chemoreceptors
   C. pCO_2 of CNS capillary blood on chemosensors of the medulla
   D. cerebrospinal fluid pH
   E. all are correct

DIRECTIONS (Questions 321–323): This section consists of a case history, followed by a series of questions. Study the history and select the **one best** answer to **each** question following it.

Case History (Questions 321–323): A 50-year-old woman enters the hospital because of cough, weight loss, and dyspnea. She was found to have a mass in her right middle lobe bronchus. On radiographic analysis the area of the right middle lobe was denser than usual and somewhat smaller in size. The following values were obtained

	Patient	Normal
Vital capacity	4.5	6 L
FRC (functional reserve capacity)	3.0	1.7 L
FEV_1 (forced expiratory volume)	2.0	4.5 L
MBC (maximum breathing capacity)	90	165 L/min
PaO_2	65	90 mm Hg
$PaCO_2$	43	38–42 mm Hg
PaO_2 during O_2 breathing	160 mm Hg	550 mm Hg
$PaCO_2$ during O_2 breathing	43 mm Hg	38–42 mm Hg

A single-breath N_2 washout test showed a progressive rise of nitrogen concentration over the course of expiration at a slope greater than normal. There was an abrupt rise in expired N_2 concentration which occurred at the point where the patient had exhaled to functional residual capacity (FRC).

To evaluate for possible surgery, a balloon-tipped catheter was placed in the right pulmonary artery (PA) and the artery was occluded by balloon inflation. The following data were obtained

Mean PA pressure	40 mm Hg
Cardiac output	4 L/min
Total pulmonary diffusion capacity	15 mL O_2/min/mm Hg

321. In this patient
  A. the arterial hypoxemia present during air breathing is caused primarily by generalized hypoventilation
  B. there is no evidence which would support the existence of an abnormally large anatomic shunt

C. an increased compliance alone could cause the abnormal FEV_1, FRC, N_2 washout
D. the vessels of the left lung are probably normal
E. a decreased compliance could explain all of the above data

322. The above data indicate
   A. the existence of a significant physiologic dead space
   B. the effective peribronchial pressure during expiration is probably lower than normal in this patient
   C. impaired diffusion does not become manifest as arterial blood hypoxemia while exercising this patient when she has had one pulmonary artery occluded
   D. a reduced ventilation/perfusion (V/P) ratio in the right middle lobe would appear as an increased physiologic shunt measured while breathing room air
   E. an anatomic shunt since this patient has a greatly reduced V/P

323. The data from this patient indicate that
   A. collapse of the right middle lobe behind an obstructing tumor can cause all the abnormalities except the N_2 washout and the reduced FRC
   B. blood flow through the partially obstructed middle lobe is reduced by the effect of alveolar hypoxia acting on the vessels. This is opposite to the effect of alveolar hypoxia in the fetal lung
   C. calculation of the physiologic shunt fraction requires knowledge of mixed systemic venous blood O_2 content in addition to the data given previously
   D. the N_2 washout curve indicates that the distribution of inspired gas, or the sequence of regional emptying, or both, are as uniform as normal in this patient
   E. there is no abnormality of respiratory function

MATCHING

DIRECTIONS (Questions 324–337): Each group of questions below consists of a set of lettered components followed by a list of numbered words or phrases. For **each** numbered word or phrase, select the **one** lettered component that is most closely associated with it. Each lettered component may be selected once, more than once, or not at all.

Questions 324–330:

- **A.** anemic hypoxia
- **B.** hypoxic hypoxia
- **C.** histotoxic hypoxia
- **D.** circulatory hypoxia

324. Breathing atmospheric air at high altitudes

325. Thromboembolism occluding a leg vein

326. Venous pO_2 higher than normal

327. Mercury poisoning of respiratory enzymes

328. Carbon monoxide poisoning of hemoglobin

329. Excessive blood loss

330. Drowning

Questions 331–337:

- **A.** apneustic center
- **B.** pneumotaxic center
- **C.** medullary respiratory center
- **D.** apneustic and pneumotaxic centers
- **E.** apneustic and medullary centers

331. Required for rhythmic breathing

332. Role seems to be similar to that of vagal afferents

333. Present in the pons

334. Center for inspiratory drive

335. Center for expiratory drive

336. Stimulated by elevated serum pCO_2

337. Ablation results in apneustic breathing or slow deep breathing

Respiratory Physiology

Answers and Discussion

265. (C) The response of the body to a low plasma pH due to a metabolic imbalance is to decrease plasma HCO_3^- by blowing off CO_2 and to excrete increased amounts of H^+ in the urine. (**Ref. 2,** pp. 673–677)

266. (D) After exercise, humans continue to use oxygen at greater than rest levels. The difference between post-exercise and resting levels of O_2 uptake is known as oxygen debt. (**Ref. 2,** pp. 625–627)

267. (B) During compensated metabolic alkalosis there is a gain of CO_2 in an attempt to return the pH toward normal. The result is increased HCO_3^-, pCO_2, and a near-normal pH. (**Ref. 2,** pp. 674–677)

268. (C) Alveolar ventilation = Respiratory volume × expired pCO_2/arterial pCO_2 (**Ref. 2,** pp. 602–604)

269. (B) During respiratory alkalosis pCO_2 decreases because CO_2 is blown off during excess ventilation with a concomitant fall in H^+ concentration. (**Ref. 2,** pp. 619, 672–673)

270. (C) Dynamic collapse of bronchioles occurs with forced expiration when the external pressure applied to the muscles of respiration exceeds the internal pressure of the bronchi. (**Ref. 2,** pp. 597–600)

271. (A) An increase in pCO_2 from the normal level of 40 mm Hg to 63 mm Hg causes a tenfold increase in alveolar ventilation. An increase in pCO_2 stimulates alveolar ventilation, not only directly but also indirectly through its effects on hydrogen ion concentration. **(Ref. 2,** pp. 615–621)

272. (C) Groups of neurons in the medulla which give rise to alternating inspiratory and expiratory activity are the fundamental source of respiratory rhythmicity. **(Ref. 2,** pp. 615–617)

273. (E) The red cell component of lung diffusion represents only 1% to 5% of the total lung resistance to diffusion of O_2. **(Ref. 2,** pp. 608–610)

274. (C) Increased pulmonary ventilation is seen in compensated metabolic acidosis. It is characterized by rapid elimination of CO_2 in an attempt to raise pH. The respiratory compensation is partial (50%–75%). **(Ref. 2,** pp. 673–677)

275. (D) CO_2 equilibrates between serum and tissues very rapidly. **(Ref. 2,** p. 635)

276. (A) The capillary pressure of 7 mm Hg is almost exactly halfway between the mean pulmonary arterial pressure of 13 mm Hg and the left atrial pressure of 2 mm Hg, indicating the arterial and venous resistances of the lungs are approximately equal. This is in marked contrast to the systemic circulation in which the arterial resistance is four to seven times as great as the venous resistance. **(Ref. 2,** pp. 604–607)

277. (A) The vital capacity is the sum of the tidal volume and the inspiratory and expiratory reserve volumes. **(Ref. 2,** pp. 594–595)

278. (A) Inspiration is an active event. Expiration during quiet breathing is a passive event. There is a tendency for the chest wall to expand outward and the lung to move inward during relaxation. The latter event is due to the elastic recoil of the lung. These forces are opposite in direction but equal in magnitude. The respiratory activity is controlled by the medulla and pons with higher influences from the cerebral cortex, as when one wants to hold their breath. **(Ref. 2,** pp. 594–595, 615–619)

279. (B) CO_2 is carried in the blood in combination with hemoglobin, as dissolved CO_2 gas, and mainly as bicarbonate. (**Ref. 2,** pp. 613–614)

280. (E) Many things influence O_2 uptake and CO_2 removal. These include stretch receptors in the lung, chemoreceptors in the arteries, and changes in metabolic activity. Due to their relative positions, the pumping of the heart exerts a mechanical action on the lung and promotes the distribution of O_2 within the lungs. Intrathoracic pressure can influence venous return and consequently cardiac output. (**Ref. 2,** pp. 608–614)

281. (B) The diaphragm is a dome-shaped muscle that flattens when contracted. This contraction increases the anteroposterior, lateral, and vertical dimensions of the thoracic cage. The positive pressure in the abdomen forces the lower ribs outward. (**Ref. 2,** pp. 595–596)

282. (D) The diaphragm is the principal muscle of respiration accounting for over two-thirds of inspired air; even more during anesthesia. Two-thirds of the fibers of the diaphragm are slow-twitch which help prevent the diaphragm from becoming fatigued. It is supplied by the phrenic nerve. (**Ref. 2,** pp. 595–596)

283. (A) The energy expended during breathing can be measured in terms of oxygen cost. This is measured at rest during normal ventilation and at increased voluntary hyperventilation. Oxygen consumption of the breathing apparatus is usually 1 mL/L or less than 5% of total body consumption of O_2. (**Ref. 2,** pp. 599–600)

284. (B) The functional residual capacity is the volume of air in the lungs at normal, end-expiratory, resting state. (**Ref. 2,** pp. 595–596)

285. (D) Total volume is the amount of air inhaled and exhaled during breathing. The maximum volume that can be inhaled from functional residual capacity is the inspiratory capacity (IC). The volume of air left at the end of normal, resting exhalation is the functional residual capacity. The volume at maximum inspiration is total lung capacity. (**Ref. 2,** pp. 595–596)

286. (C) Elastin and collagen give lung tissue its resilience. Elastin allows stretching while collagen prevents overstretching.

Emphysema is a disease that degrades elastin and collagen as well as the alveolar walls. The result is an increase in the distensibility of the lung. (**Ref. 2,** pp. 597–598)

287. (**E**)   Chest wall expansion represents 70% of total lung capacity if opposed by the lung. However, at values greater than 70% the chest wall recoils inward; at volumes less than 70% it recoils outward. (**Ref. 2,** pp. 594–596)

288. (**A**)   Flow rate is directly proportional to the driving pressure, varies inversely with the length of the tube and viscosity, and is to the fourth power of the tube radius. Flow is not always laminar. (**Ref. 2,** pp. 531–532)

289. (**E**)   The parabolic profile of laminar flow is characteristic of both air and fluid. However, gas molecules can move laterally and collide to form eddys much more readily. Gas flow rate varies with the square root of the driving pressure, but for all practical purposes is independent of density. (**Ref. 2,** pp. 530–532)

290. (**E**)   Resistance is very high for nasal passage but air flow decreases as cross-sectional area increases, which is what happens with each successive branching of the bronchi. Therefore, air flow resistance decreases with each successive branching. (**Ref. 2,** pp. 597–598)

291. (**B**)   At the beginning of forced expiration, just as the lung volume begins to decrease, lung elastic recoil decreases along with the transmural pressure. The intrathoracic airways narrow, which increases airway resistance. (**Ref. 2,** pp. 597–602)

292. (**B**)   During a maximal inspiratory effort, the pleural pressure is subatmospheric. The muscles of inspiration diminish in their force generation according to length tension properties of muscle. This results in a progressive reduction in air flow. The transmural pressure is large. (**Ref. 2,** pp. 594–596)

293. (**C**)   Approximately 60% of the CO_2 in venous blood is in the form of bicarbonate, with 7% in the dissolved state and 23% in the carbamino form. (**Ref. 2,** pp. 613–614)

294. (B) Increased carbon dioxide, 2,3-DPG and temperature, and decreased pH shift the curve to the right and down releasing O_2 from hemoglobin at any given alveolar pO_2. (**Ref. 2** pp. 608–610)

295. (D) Intrapulmonary pressure is determined by airway resistance and direction of airflow. (**Ref. 2,** pp. 597–599)

296. (C) A major role of respiration is the removal of CO_2. A low pCO_2 results in a decrease in ventilation. (**Ref. 2,** pp. 617–621)

297. (E) Increased body temperature and serum pCO_2, decreased serum pH, and joint movement will produce hyperpnea. The higher centers in the central nervous system also have an influence for the respiratory increases. (**Ref. 2,** pp. 619–621, 625–627)

298. (B) The diffusion coefficient of O_2 in tissues is 20 times lower than that for CO_2 because the diffusion coefficient for the transfer of each gas through the respiratory membrane depends on its solubility in the membrane and inversely on the square root of its molecular weight. (**Ref. 2,** pp. 608–610)

299. (A) Sensory input from the vagus nerve to the respiratory centers in the brain stem is necessary for normal rhythm rate and depth of respiration. (**Ref. 2,** pp. 616–617)

300. (E) Severe gastric vomiting from deep in the GI system will result in a metabolic acidosis with CO_2 accumulation and corresponding increases in bicarbonate; respiration will occur to compensate for the acidosis. (**Ref. 2,** pp. 673–677)

301. (C) The factors listed illustrate the importance of hemoglobin as a reserve for O_2. (**Ref. 2,** pp. 608–610)

302. (E) The release of O_2 by hemoglobin in vascular beds is facilitated by low pO_2, low pH, high temperature, and high pCO_2. (**Ref. 2,** p. 608–610)

303. (D) Carbon monoxide has a very high affinity for binding to a specific site on the hemoglobin molecule. (**Ref. 2,** pp. 633–634)

304. (E) The Hering-Breuer reflexes result in inhibition of inspiration when the lungs are inflated and excitation of inspiration when the lungs are deflated. **(Ref. 2,** pp. 622–623)

305. (B) The total O_2 in the blood will be largely determined by how much hemoglobin is present. Hence, when red cell numbers decrease in anemia, total oxygen goes down. **(Ref. 2,** pp. 608–610)

306. (C) The compliance of a lung is calculated by dividing ΔV by ΔP. For a lung showing a volume change of 1 L with a pressure change of 5 cm of H_2O, the compliance would be .20. **(Ref. 2,** pp. 597–598)

307. (B) If an alveolus has perfusion without ventilation, the O_2 in the alveolus will be depleted until it is at the level of mixed venous blood. At this point the blood flowing around the alveolus will appear as if it had passed through an arteriovenous shunt. **(Ref. 2,** pp. 631–632)

308. (A) The ventilation perfusion ratio is determined by dividing the total alveolar ventilation by the cardiac output. **(Ref. 2,** pp. 631–632)

309. (C) The pontine respiratory center contains both the apneustic center, which, if stimulated, will cause apneustic breathing, and the pneumotaxic center, which is largely concerned with controlling the rate of respiration. **(Ref. 2,** pp. 616–617)

310. (D) The presentation of 100% O_2 to a patient with a prominent carotid body drive (i.e., a low arterial O_2) often results in respiratory arrest. **(Ref. 2,** pp. 617–619)

311. (D) Pulmonary emphysema is a degenerative disorder leading to disruption of alveolar septa and pulmonary fibrosis with a decrease in efficiency of alveolar ventilation. In chronically and severely hypoxic persons, the slowly adapting chemoreceptors provide not only reflex activation of the respiratory centers, but an arousal mechanism for higher functions such as consciousness. **(Ref. 2,** p. 633)

312. (E) The work of breathing can be broken up into a series of elements including the work against inertia, the work against elastic elements, and the work to overcome airway resistance. (**Ref. 2,** pp. 599–600)

313. (A) Dyspnea is defined as the sensation of inadequate or distressful breathing. (**Ref. 2,** p. 627)

314. (E) Most of the volume change in the lung occurs in the respiratory bronchioles. (**Ref. 2,** pp. 591–594)

315. (B) The curves shown in Figure 13 demonstrate several things. At increasing pHs, there is an increased affinity of hemoglobin for oxygen, and that the affinity of hemoglobin for oxygen changes as the pO_2 varies. (**Ref. 2,** pp. 609–610)

316. (C) Higher temperature, concentration of 2,3-DPG (2,3-diphosphoglycerate), and pCO_2 all shift hemoglobin oxygen saturation curves to the right. (**Ref. 2,** pp. 609–610)

317. (B) The major action of the diaphragm is to decrease the intrathoracic pressure when it contracts. (**Ref. 2,** pp. 595–596)

318. (A) Lung surfactant is a phospholipid that adjusts the surface tension of the air liquid interface of the alveoli in order to decrease the likelihood of alveolar collapse during expiration. The surface tension of the alveoli is maintained at a relatively constant and low level of lung surfactant that is concentrated as the alveoli shrink during expiration. (**Ref. 2,** pp. 598–599)

319. (E) The activities of gas molecules in the lung are governed by the gas laws.

320. (E) The control systems for respiration include all the factors. The most sensitive factor appears to be the pCO_2 of the blood. (**Ref. 2,** pp. 615–620)

321. (C) The patient's vital capacity is not that low. An anatomic shunt would be evident if the ventilation/perfusion (V/P) ratio were greatly reduced, which it is not in this patient. In addition, the vessels of the lung are abnormal because the patient's cardiac output is normal. Hence, a great proportion of the output must be going to the lungs. However, an increased compliance can cause the abnormalities seen above. (**Ref. 2,** pp. 597–598)

322. (D) Although there is no real anatomic shunt (because the V/P ratio is not greatly reduced), the breathing of room air results in an apparent physiologic (not anatomic) shunt. (**Ref. 2,** pp. 631–632)

323. (C) The shunting of mixed venous pulmonary arterial blood around alveolar capillaries and directly into the pulmonary veins can be detected by a 100% oxygen breathing test because the level of oxygenation of mixed venous blood would be directly proportional to the amount of blood that is shunted. (**Ref. 2,** pp. 631–632)

324. (B) Atmospheric air at high altitudes has low partial pressures of all gases, hence the pO_2 is lowered sufficiently to give hypoxic hypoxia. (**Ref. 2,** pp. 628–630)

325. (D) The reduction in blood flow due to a thromboembolism occluding a leg vein will give rise to stagnantoxia or circulatory hypoxia. (**Ref. 2,** p. 634)

326. (C) A venous pO_2 higher than normal would indicate that the perfused tissue is unable to utilize the O_2 being presented to it. This is usually classified as histotoxic hypoxia. (**Ref. 2,** p. 634)

327. (C) If the respiratory enzymes of a tissue are poisoned by mercury they will be unable to utilize O_2 and a histotoxic hypoxia will result. (**Ref. 2,** p. 634)

328. (A) Carbon monoxide poisoning removes some of the hemoglobin available for O_2 transport. This results in an anemic anoxia. (**Ref. 2,** pp. 633–634)

329. (A) Excessive blood loss also removes some of the hemoglobin available for transport and results in an anemic anoxia. (**Ref. 2,** p. 633)

330. (B) Immersion of the head in water cuts off the supply of fresh air to the lungs and results in an hypoxic hypoxia. (**Ref. 2,** pp. 628–631)

331. (C) The medullary respiratory center is responsible for alternating inspiration that is the essential activity of breathing. (**Ref. 2,** pp. 615–617)

332. (B) The role of the pneumotaxic center is to control the rate of respiration, and is similar in action to the vagal afferents. (**Ref. 2,** pp. 615–617)

333. (D) Both the apneustic and pneumotaxic centers are found in the pons. (**Ref. 2,** pp. 615–617)

334. (E) The apneustic and medullary centers supply the drive for inspiration. (**Ref. 2,** pp. 615–617)

335. (C) The medullary respiratory center is responsible for supplying the drive for expiration. (**Ref. 2,** pp. 615–617)

336. (E) Both the apneustic center and the medullary centers are activated by elevated serum pCO_2. (**Ref. 2,** pp. 615–617)

337. (B) Ablation of the pneumotaxic center releases the apneustic center from its influence. This results in apneustic or slow deep breathing. (**Ref. 2,** pp. 615–617)

5

Renal Physiology

MULTIPLE CHOICE

DIRECTIONS (Questions 338–381): Each of the questions or incomplete statements below is followed by five suggested answers or completions. Select the **one** that is **best** in each case.

338. The volume of plasma needed each minute to supply a substance at the rate at which it is excreted in the urine is known as the
  A. diffusion constant of the substance
  B. clearance of the substance
  C. extraction ratio of the substance
  D. tubular mass of the substance
  E. filtration rate of the substance

339. Total renal blood flow of both human kidneys is what fraction of the resting cardiac output?
  A. 5%
  B. 10%
  C. 25%
  D. 40%
  E. 50%

340. An increase in the osmolality of the extracellular compartment will
  A. stimulate the volume and osmoreceptors, and inhibit ADH secretion
  B. inhibit the volume and osmoreceptors, and stimulate ADH secretion
  C. inhibit the volume and osmoreceptors, and inhibit ADH secretion
  D. stimulate the volume and osmoreceptors, and stimulate ADH secretion
  E. cause no change in ADH secretion

341. Which of the following combinations of data would lead you to suspect that a patient had the "syndrome of inappropriate antidiuretic hormone secretion" (SIADH)?

	pOsm mOsm/kg	pNa mEq/L	mUOsm mOsm/kg
A.	286	138	627
B.	263	126	52
C.	286	138	177
D.	263	126	426
E.	300	144	100

P = plasma, U = urine

342. If the renal plasma flow is 600 mL plasma/min and the hematocrit is 40%, what is the renal blood flow (in mL/min)?
  A. 1500
  B. 1000
  C. 960
  D. 1200
  E. 1800

343. The normal human glomerular filtration rate (GFR) is approximately (in mL/min)
  A. 25
  B. 50
  C. 125
  D. 300
  E. 500

344. The role of the kidney in homeostasis may include which of the following?
   A. Secretion of certain hormones, such as angiotensin II, prostaglandins, and kinins in the regulation of blood pressure
   B. Regulation of extracellular fluid composition
   C. Regulation of red blood cell formation
   D. Secretion of erythropoietin
   E. All are correct

345. Body fluid compartments
   A. do not include bone or cartilage matrices
   B. account for less than 33% of total body water
   C. fluctuate in size in response to environmental stress or disease
   D. account for 40% of total body mass
   E. A and C are correct

346. Which of the following is(are) true concerning the various fluid compartments of the body?
   A. Total body water and the fluid volumes of each compartment change very little from day to day
   B. Movement of water (loss or gain) is in proportion to the volumes of each compartment
   C. Ions and their distribution have no effect on the volume of fluid compartments
   D. In a steady-state condition, osmotic activity is very different for various body compartments
   E. B and D are correct

347. The flow of fluid through the kidney
   A. requires an arterial blood supply via the afferent arteriole
   B. begins by entering a filtering unit called Bowman's capsule
   C. passes through the ducts of Bellini before exiting from the kidney
   D. begins in the proximal convoluted tubule by filtration, followed by reabsorption and secretion of the filtrate
   E. A, B, and C are correct

348. Which is a feature of the glomerulus?
  A. Podocyte
  B. Fenestrated epithelium
  C. Slit membrane
  D. Foot processes
  E. All are correct

349. Which of the following is(are) true regarding the Starling hypothesis for capillary exchange?
  A. Requires knowing the protein concentration in the proximal tubular fluid
  B. Can only be estimated for the kidney as a whole
  C. Describes how fast fluid crosses the glomerulus under a given filtration pressure
  D. Is the product of coefficient K divided by the algebraic sum of the glomerular capillary hydrostatic, proximal tubular hydrostatic, glomerular capillary oncotic, and proximal tubular fluid oncotic pressures
  E. A and C are correct

350. Which of the following is true regarding glomerular filtration rate (GFR)-capillary flow?
  A. At higher capillary flow rates, the net filtration pressure is reduced thereby lowering the GFR
  B. At higher capillary flow rates, the plasma oncotic pressure is lower, net filtration pressure is elevated, and GFR increases
  C. GFR remains relatively constant because the mean hydrostatic capillary pressure remains unaltered
  D. When flow is increased the plasma oncotic pressure increases more over a given distance along the capillary
  E. B and D are correct

351. Which of the following does not increase the filtration coefficient K?
  A. Prostaglandins
  B. Norepinephrine (a vasoconstrictor)
  C. Angiotensin II
  D. Acetylcholine (a vasodilator)
  E. All are correct

352. Which of the following classes of molecules are transported by the renal epithelia?
A. Organic bases
B. Aliphatic acids
C. Aromatic acids
D. Monovalent and polyvalent ions
E. All are correct

353. Processes involved in the transport of materials across the tubular epithelium are dependent upon
A. size of the molecules
B. concentration gradient
C. lipid solubility
D. charge
E. all are correct

354. Characteristics of active transport systems include
A. molecular specificity
B. insensitivity to inhibitors
C. saturation at low concentrations
D. transport rate lower than normally would be predicted for a given lipid solubility and size of a molecule
E. A and C are correct

355. Plasma threshold of a substance
A. is descriptive of a gradient-time system
B. means that over a small range of plasma concentrations excretion varies linearly
C. is descriptive of molecules that display tubular transport maximum (T_m) type characteristics
D. is the minimal plasma concentration at which reabsorption begins
E. A and C are correct

356. Gradient-time system characteristics include
A. no evidence of plasma threshold
B. excretion varies linearly
C. A and B are correct
D. excretion remains constant over a wide range of filtration rates
E. all are correct

357. Renal function can be tested by infusing a secreted dye at progressively faster rates until saturation is achieved. Analyzing urine under these conditions
  A. yields information on cardiovascular as well as tubular function
  B. yields information on cardiovascular function
  C. yields information on tubular function
  D. yields information on tubular function and tubular transport capacity
  E. all are correct

358. According to the equation for net tubular transport rate (TR = filtration rate − excretion rate) if the transport rate is positive
  A. secretion must have taken place
  B. reabsorption must have taken place
  C. excretion rate is in excess of filtration rate
  D. solute must have been added to the glomerular filtrate
  E. B and D are correct

359. The loops of Henle of the outer cortical nephrons
  A. do not contribute to the medullary osmotic gradient
  B. are functionally unimportant in the renal conservation of sodium and water
  C. do not participate in the urinary diluting mechanism
  D. do not play any important role in overall renal function and are simply unimportant vestiges of evolutionary development
  E. A and C are correct

360. In active transport, there must be
  A. presence of carrier molecule
  B. binding of solute to some membrane component
  C. energy required for transport
  D. directional sites in membrane pores
  E. A, B, and C are correct

361. Under normal conditions in humans, the colloid osmotic pressure of the blood at the capillary level
  A. is due primarily to presence of diffusible crystalloids
  B. is balanced by capillary oncotic pressure
  C. is balanced by capillary hydrostatic pressure

D. tends to inhibit the diffusion of appropriate substances for the nutritive needs of cells

E. A and C are correct

362. For those substances that are actively reabsorbed, the maximal amount that can be transported per unit time by the kidney tubules

A. depends on the maximum rate at which the transport mechanism itself operates

B. requires specific transport systems for each substance transported

C. is termed the tubular transport maximum

D. is dependent upon tubular load

E. A, B, and C are correct

363. Clearance ratios greater than 1 are most likely seen with substances which are

A. neither secreted nor absorbed

B. reabsorbed

C. secreted

D. bound to tubular proteins

E. none are correct

364. Solute particles move from the plasma of the renal glomerulus to the fluid in the Bowman's capsule by

A. bulk flow

B. active transport

C. diffusion

D. renal flow

E. A and C are correct

365. Ammonia produced by the kidneys comes mainly from

A. glycine

B. glutamine

C. leucine

D. alanine

E. B and D are correct

366. Polyuria (diuresis), which occurs in the diabetic with a GFR = 120 mL/min and blood sugar level = 350 mg%, is indicative of

A. losses of water and sodium which can be prevented by administration of antidiuretic hormone (ADH) and an aldosterone-like mineralocorticoid

B. diuresis due to reduced active transport of sodium out of the tubule because of diminished activity of the sodium pump

C. a cellular and extracellular hydration due to water retention of the glucose; hence diuresis is "never" observed in a diabetic individual

D. an osmotic diuresis due to glucosuria and the water loss will exceed "salt" loss

E. B and D are correct

367. The "renal plasma threshold" for glucose will be decreased by

A. an increase in glucose T_m

B. a decrease in glomerular filtration rate

C. a decrease in tubular reabsorption

D. an increase in the slope of the glucose reabsorbtion curve

E. A and C are correct

368. The tonicity of the urine as it enters the renal collecting duct may be

A. isotonic

B. hypotonic or isotonic, but never hypertonic

C. hypotonic

D. hypertonic

E. hypertonic or isotonic, but never hypotonic

369. Extracellular dehydration results in

A. inhibition of the volume and osmoreceptors and increased ADH secretion

B. stimulation of the volume and osmoreceptors and increased ADH secretion

C. inhibition of the volume and osmoreceptors and decreased ADH secretion

D. decreased extracellular osmolality

E. B and D are correct

370. Of the following, which are **CORRECTLY** defined or described?
  - **A.** Filtration fraction: glomerular filtration rate divided by renal plasma flow
  - **B.** Tubular maximum secretion: has a finite upper limit though exhibits a phenomenon analogous to the threshold phenomenon for reabsorption
  - **C.** Clearance ratio: renal clearance of one substance divided by the clearance of another substance
  - **D.** Effective renal plasma flow: volume of plasma flow supplied to the entire renal tissue
  - **E.** A, B, and C are correct

371. The juxtaglomerular apparatus
  - **A.** includes a long loop of Henle that dips into the medulla
  - **B.** participates in the control of aldosterone secretion through the renin-angiotensin system
  - **C.** is involved in maintaining the normal balance of calcium in the body
  - **D.** functions as a sphincter around the distal tubules
  - **E.** B and D are correct

372. About 4 to 6 days after you place a "normal" patient on a low sodium diet to reduce his or her weight, which of the following will be observed?
  - **A.** Plasma renin and aldosterone are below normal
  - **B.** Plasma renin and aldosterone are above normal
  - **C.** Plasma sodium concentration is below normal
  - **D.** Plasma sodium concentration is above normal
  - **E.** B and D are correct

373. You have two patients (each weighing 80 kg), one of whom you give 1000 mL of distilled water (subject A), while the other you give 1000 mL of isotonic saline (subject B). Both drink the fluid within the same length of time. Correct statements regarding subjects A and B include
  - **A.** subject A will have a smaller urinary output within 2 hours after the fluid intake
  - **B.** subject B has the greater increase in plasma volume
  - **C.** subject A has a greater change in plasma osmolality
  - **D.** subject B has the greater change in urine osmolality
  - **E.** none are correct

374. The substance(s) which makes up the greatest part of the reabsorptive "load" in the renal tubule is (are)
A. urea
B. glucose
C. potassium
D. sodium
E. glycine

375. The renal "countercurrent" mechanism is dependent upon the anatomic arrangement of the
A. loop of Henle
B. glomerulus
C. vasa recta
D. proximal tubule
E. A and C are correct

376. Secretion of aldosterone will result from
A. low extracellular potassium
B. low extracellular volume
C. high extracellular sodium
D. smoking, agitation, and stress
E. B and D are correct

377. Aldosterone secretion is controlled by levels of
A. angiotensin II
B. plasma calcium
C. plasma bicarbonate
D. ADH
E. A and C are correct

378. Figure 14 graphically represents the data collected from a patient following the oral ingestion of a solution. The solution probably was
A. 5% NaCl
B. .9% NaCl
C. .9% KCl
D. water
E. 15% glucose

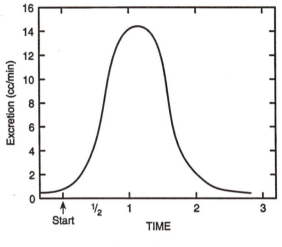

Figure 14

DIRECTIONS (Questions 379–381): This section consists of a situation, followed by a series of questions. Study the situation, and select the one **best** answer to **each** question following it.

The following data were obtained in an 80-kg male patient during renal clearance tests

---

Para-aminohippuric acid (PAH) concentration in plasma	.3 ug/mL
PAH concentration in urine	90.0 ug/mL
Inulin concentration in plasma	10.0 ug/mL
Inulin concentration in urine	.6 mg/mL
pO_4 concentration in plasma	.5 uM/mL
pO_4 concentration in urine	1.0 uM/mL
Hematocrit	40%
Urine flow	2 mL/min

---

379. The glomerular filtration rate in mL/min is

    A. 120

    B. 150

    C. 180

    D. 240

    E. 400

380. The renal plasma flow in mL/min is
 A. 100
 B. 300
 C. 600
 D. 900
 E. 1200

381. The renal blood flow in mL/min is
 A. 100
 B. 300
 C. 600
 D. 1000
 E. 1200

MATCHING

DIRECTIONS (Questions 382–414): Each group of questions below consists of a set of lettered components, followed by a list of numbered words or phrases. For **each** numbered word or phrase, select the **one** lettered component that is most closely associated with it. Each lettered component may be selected once, more than once, or not at all.

Questions 382–387 (Figure 15):

 A. site A
 B. site B
 C. site C
 D. site D
 E. site E

In Figure 15 the site(s) at which there is the greatest or highest

382. Net fluid transport is

383. Dilution of solutes is

384. Amino acid reabsorption is

385. Na^+ reabsorption is

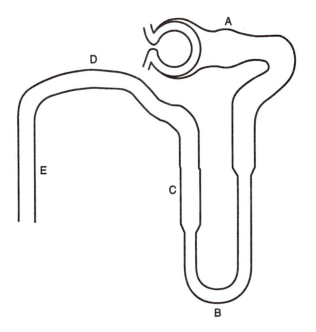

Figure 15

386. Concentration of solutes is

387. Active Na^+/Cl^- transport is

Questions 388–395:

    A. increases from the normal average value
    B. decreases from the normal average value
    C. no change from the normal average value

A patient develops an increase in mean systemic blood pressure and blood volume. Indicate how the increased blood pressure and volume would affect the following

388. Secretion of the juxtaglomerular cells of the kidney

389. Angiotensin secretion

390. Adrenal cortex stimulation

391. Aldosterone secretion

392. ADH secretion

393. Na^+ reabsorption

394. K^+ reabsorption

395. H_2O reabsorption

Questions 396–398:

    A. increases from the normal average value
    B. decreases from the normal average value
    C. no change from the normal average value

During the early hypotensive phase of hemorrhagic shock, indicate how the alterations with this early shock affect the following

396. The hematocrit

397. The cardiac output

398. Peripheral resistance

Questions 399–401:

    A. increases from the normal average value
    B. decreases from the normal average value
    C. no change from the normal average value

During the irreversible phase of hemorrhagic shock

399. Plasma protein concentration

400. Precapillary to post-capillary resistance ratio

401. Mean arterial blood pressure

Questions 402–406:

    A. 4%–5% of lean body mass
    B. 12%–15% of lean body mass
    C. 20%–24% of lean body mass
    D. 40%–50% of lean body mass
    E. 60%–70% of lean body mass

402. Total body water

403. Interstitial compartment water

404. Intracellular water content

405. Vascular (plasma) water content

406. Extracellular fluid

Questions 407–414:

    A. increases from the normal average value
    B. decreases from the normal average value
    C. no change from the normal average value

407. pCO_2 of the plasma during respiratory acidosis

408. HCO_3^- concentration of the plasma during respiratory acidosis

409. pCO_2 of the plasma during respiratory alkalosis

410. HCO_3^- concentration of the plasma during respiratory alkalosis

411. pCO_2 of the plasma during metabolic acidosis

412. HCO_3^- concentration of the plasma during metabolic acidosis

413. pCO_2 of the plasma during metabolic alkalosis

414. HCO_3^- concentration of the plasma during metabolic alkalosis

Renal Physiology

Answers and Discussion

338. (B) Renal clearance is defined as the volume of plasma containing the amount of a substance that is excreted in the urine. (**Ref. 2,** pp. 645–650)

339. (C) Renal blood flow through both kidneys accounts for one-fourth of the cardiac output. (**Ref. 2,** pp. 645–646)

340. (D) ADH is one of the primary mechanisms for the control of plasma osmolality. (**Ref. 2,** pp. 221–222)

341. (D) When plasma osmolality and plasma sodium are low, there should be an excretion of water. If, however, the urine osmolality remains high in spite of the low plasma values, inappropriate ADH secretion should be considered. (**Ref. 2,** pp. 221–222)

342. (B) Renal blood flow = Renal plasma flow/(1 − hematocrit), thus RBF = 600/(1 − .40) = 1000 mL blood/min. (**Ref. 2,** p. 486)

343. (C) According to measurements made with inulin, the GFR in the male is about 125 mL/min. In the female it is about 10% less. To compare the GFRs in individuals of various sizes it is customary to normalize the values to that of an ideal person with a body surface of 1.73 cm^2. (**Ref. 2,** p. 648)

344. (E) The function of the kidney is to regulate the extracellular fluid composition thereby providing a constant environment for the cells of the body to exist. The role of the kidney in the regulation of extracellular fluids and their composition is achieved through neural and humoral means. These mechanisms include secretion of angiotensin II, prostaglandins, and kinins—hormones essential to the regulation of blood pressure, as well as filtration, reabsorption, and secretion of the various components of the body fluids. Erythropoietin, another hormone secreted by the kidney, helps regulate red cell formation. (**Ref. 2,** p. 641)

345. (C) Total body water volume is separated into several compartments, the principle compartments being extracellular, intracellular, and interstitial. Sixty percent of total body weight can be attributed to the water content of the body. This includes water which is inaccessible [i.e., bound up in cartilage, tendon, and the matrices of bone (approximately 10%)]. This latter fluid compartment is termed the transcellular compartment. (**Ref. 2,** pp. 670–671)

346. (B) Fluid volumes as well as total body water can fluctuate greatly over the course of a day. However, osmotic activity of each compartment remains relatively balanced due to the proportional movement of fluid from each compartment. The Donnan effect explains the effect ion distribution has on fluid compartment size. (**Ref. 2,** pp. 670–671)

347. (A) The flow of fluid through the kidney begins with the primary filtration in the glomerulus inside Bowman's capsule (not in the proximal tubules). The blood is supplied to the glomerulus via the afferent arteriole, passes through the glomerular capillaries, and exits through the efferent arteriole. This filtrate flows through a highly convoluted section called the proximal convoluted tubule. The tubule extends toward or into the medulla forming a hairpin turn called the loop of Henle with its descending and ascending loops. From the ascending loop fluid enters the distal convoluted tubule and from there into collecting ducts. The urine exits the kidney through small pores called the ducts of Bellini. (**Ref. 2,** pp. 641–644)

348. (E) The podocytes are specialized epithelial cells which are a continuation of the proximal tubule endothelium. The fenestrated endothelium is a continuation of the arterioles supplying the glomerulus. The slit membrane spans two podocytes and acts as a molecular sieve. The foot processes are extensions of the podocytes. (**Ref. 2,** pp. 641–644)

349. **(A)** Knowing the protein concentration in the proximal tubular fluid allows one to apply the Starling hypothesis for capillary exchange. The algebraic expression is the product of the coefficient times the sum of the glomerular capillary hydrostatic, proximal tubular hydrostatic, glomerular capillary oncotic, and proximal tubular fluid oncotic pressures. K is a coefficient that describes how fast fluid crosses the glomerulus under a given pressure. Values for K can be estimated for a single glomerulus or for an entire kidney. (**Ref. 2,** pp. 537–538)

350. **(B)** Plasma oncotic pressure rises significantly along the length of the glomerular capillary relative to the capillary flow rate. At lower capillary flow rates, the plasma spends more time at a particular location. Thus, it has a chance to increase more over a given distance traveling along the capillary. Therefore, at higher flow rates the oncotic pressure does not increase as quickly and the hydrostatic pressure is higher, which increases the GFR. (**Ref. 2,** pp. 647–650)

351. **(E)** Angiotensin II, bradykinin, and prostaglandins all decrease the filtration coefficient. Curiously, vasodilators, such as acetylcholine, and vasoconstrictors, such as norepinephrine, also decrease the filtration coefficient for reasons that are not yet clear. (**Ref. 2,** pp. 646–647)

352. **(E)** Typical classes of molecules transported by the renal epithelia include monovalent and polyvalent ions such as Na^+, Cl^-, and pO_4^- and calcium, respectively. Aromatic and aliphatic acids such as penicillin and pyruvate, respectively, and organic bases such as thiamine are also transported. Large molecules such as glucose require a special transport system. (**Ref. 2,** pp. 650–654)

353. **(E)** All are intrinsic characteristics of the material being transported which affects the transportability of that material. In other words, size, charge, solubility, and concentration are factors that affect transport. Small uncharged molecules traverse rather easily. Large molecules traverse more slowly or require special transport mechanisms. (**Ref. 2,** pp. 28–31)

354. **(A)** Active transport, to some extent, follows the kinetics of enzyme activity. Active transport systems are sensitive to inhibitors and compete for similar molecules despite their molecular specificity. They become saturated at high concentrations. (**Ref. 2,** pp. 28–31)

355. **(C)** Using glucose, which displays T_m characteristics as an example, increasing plasma glucose concentration from zero produces no change in excretion initially. However, once glucose reaches a plasma level of about 200 mg/dL of plasma, excretion begins to rise curvilinearly. This curvilinear range is termed the splay. Concentrations above the splay imply that the system is saturated, the difference between filtration and reabsorption is a constant, and any increase in filtration directly increases excretion. (**Ref. 2,** pp. 652–653)

356. **(C)** It is assumed that the gradient-time system has a lower affinity relative to plasma concentrations. Therefore, it does not become saturated. Using sodium as an example, 67% of the sodium filtered is reabsorbed over a wide range of filtration rates. Since excretion varies linearly over a wide range of plasma concentrations, there is no evidence of a threshold. (**Ref. 2,** pp. 657–660)

357. **(E)** Analysis of urine under saturation conditions gives an estimate of the tubular transport capacity. This transport capacity also depends on renal blood flow. As a result, this type of testing yields information on cardiovascular as well as tubular function. (**Ref. 2,** pp. 650–660)

358. **(B)** According to the equation net transport rate = filtration rate − excretion rate, if the transport rate is negative, then excretion rate is greater than filtration rate. In other words some secretion must have taken place (solute has been added to glomerular filtrate). On the other hand, if less material appears in the final urine than originally had been filtered, then reabsorption has taken place. (**Ref. 2,** pp. 650–660)

359. **(A)** The countercurrent mechanism responsible for the secretion of hyperosmotic urine requires the penetration of loops of Henle into the renal medulla for the development of a medullary osmotic gradient. The loops of the outer cortical nephron do not descend into the inner medulla. (**Ref. 2,** pp. 657–660)

360. (E) An active transport system must have energy, a carrier system, and some method for sequestering the transported system when it reaches the cell membrane. (**Ref. 2,** pp. 22–27)

361. (C) The functional capillary pressure is about 17 mm Hg while the tissue pressure is nearly 0. The presence of nondiffusible (at best poorly diffusible) proteins in the capillaries exerts an osmotic pressure equal but opposite to the capillary hydrostatic pressure. This osmotic pressure due to the presence of these proteins is called the colloid osmotic or oncotic pressure. (**Ref. 2,** pp. 537–538)

362. (E) The tubular transport maximum (T_m) is the maximal amount of a given material that can be transported across the tubular membrane per unit time. This transport maximum depends largely on the speed at which the transport mechanism itself can operate. Since substances are reabsorbed or secreted, T_m is independent of tubular load, which is the amount of substance filtered through the glomerulus each minute. However, the relationship between tubular load and T_m will affect final urine concentration of the substance. (**Ref. 2,** pp. 650–654)

363. (C) The ratio of the amount of a substance filtered to the amount of that same substance cleared in the urine is the clearance ratio for that substance. When secretion is involved, one sees clearance ratios greater than 1. With reabsorption, clearance ratios are less than 1. For substances that are neither secreted nor absorbed, clearance = GFR. (**Ref. 2,** p. 660)

364. (A) Movement of water molecules through the glomerulus is often greater than that accounted for by simple net diffusion. This "streaming" of molecules is termed bulk flow. Bulk flow is a characteristic of extremely permeable membranes such as those found in the renal glomerulus. (**Ref. 2,** pp. 641–644)

365. (B) The major fraction of urinary ammonia is derived from the amide nitrogen of glutamine. (**Ref. 2,** p. 662)

366. (D) Polyuria associated with a high blood glucose level is an osmotic event that will affect water loss to a much greater extent than electrolyte loss. (**Ref** 2, pp. 658–659, 666)

367. (C) The renal plasma threshold for the appearance of glucose in the urine will be decreased by an increase in glomerular filtration rate, a decrease in glucose T_m, decreased tubular reabsorption of glucose, and a decrease in the slope of the glucose reabsorbtion curve. (**Ref. 2**, pp. 652–653)

368. (B) Because of the osmotic gradient from the outer cortex to the inner medulla of the kidney, urine, as it enters the collecting ducts, only can be hypotonic, or at best isotonic, but not hypertonic. (**Ref. 2**, pp. 656–657)

369. (B) An increase in extracellular fluid osmolality (excess Na^+ and its associated anions) stimulates the osmoreceptors within the supraoptic nuclei of the hypothalamus. Impulses from the nuclei traverse through the pituitary stalk into the posterior pituitary gland promoting the release of ADH. In addition, the extracellular fluid osmolality increases and by definition means that extracellular fluid volume is less than normal. The reduction of stretch with the atria which follows thereby reduces nerve signals into the brain to cause an increase in ADH secretion. (**Ref. 2**, pp. 221–224)

370. (E) All are correct except D. Effective renal plasma flow describes the delivery of plasma to the peritubular capillaries. (**Ref. 2**, pp. 645–650)

371. (B) The juxtaglomerular apparatus found in juxtamedullary nephrons which have long loops of Henle is important in body sodium homeostasis and aldosterone secretion. It is composed of the macula densa, extraglomerular mesengeal cells, and granular cells. (**Ref. 2**, pp. 655–660)

372. (B) As soon as an individual is placed on a low sodium diet, the normal mechanisms of the body will attempt to conserve the sodium available. Hence, renin and aldosterone will be high and plasma sodium concentration will be about normal. (**Ref. 2**, pp. 663–664)

373. (C) A subject ingesting distilled water will have a rapid decrease in plasma and urine osmolality because of dilution. In addition, the individual receiving distilled water will have a more rapid increase in urine production because the system controlling plasma osmolality works more rapidly than the system controlling plasma volume. (**Ref. 2,** pp. 658–660)

374. (**D**) Sodium represents by far the largest portion of tubular reabsorption. (**Ref. 2,** p. 663)

375. (**E**) The excretion of hypertonic urine utilizing the countercurrent multiplier mechanism depends on the anatomic arrangement of the loop of Henle, the vasa recta, and collecting ducts going through the hypertonic medulla in order to allow the urine to become concentrated by equilibrating (in the presence of ADH) with the medullary interstitial fluid. (**Ref. 2,** pp. 657–659)

376. (**E**) High extracellular potassium, low extracellular volume, sodium, smoking, agitation, and stress all stimulate aldosterone secretion. (**Ref. 2,** pp. 663–664)

377. (**A**) Angiotensin II as well as total plasma volume are potent signals for activation of the zona glomerulosa to release aldosterone. (**Ref. 2,** pp. 663–664)

378. (**D**) The normal rate of urine flow is 1 mL/min with an osmolality of around 1000 mOsm/kg H_2O. If 1 L of water is ingested, the urine flow increases within 20 min and peaks within 1 hour. The urine osmolality is inversely related to the rate of urine flow. Since both GFR and rate of solute excretion remain the same, the change in water excretion results from differences in tubular reabsorption of water, and hence, is due to a decreased secretion of ADH. (**Ref. 2,** pp. 658–660)

379. (**A**) The glomerular filtration rate can be calculated from the clearance in inulin since it is neither excreted nor absorbed by the renal tubules.

$$GFR = \text{inulin concentration in urine} \times \text{urine flow/} \\ \text{concentration of inulin in plasma}$$

(**Ref. 2,** p. 647)

380. (C) Renal plasma flow can be calculated if a material is available which is not metabolized by the kidney and if the amount in the urine and loss per liter of plasma are known.

Renal plasma flow = amount of urine per unit time/loss/L plasma

(Ref. 2, p. 645)

381. (D) Renal blood flow can be calculated from renal plasma flow and the hematocrit. **(Ref. 2,** p. 645)

382. (A) Normally, more than 99% of the filtered water is reabsorbed as it passes through the tubules, of which 65% (55 mL/min of the cleared 12 L/min) is reabsorbed in the proximal portion passively by osmosis. As a substance is reabsorbed (passively or actively) the concentration within the proximal tubule decreases causing water to move out of the tubule by osmosis. **(Ref. 2,** pp. 654–660)

383. (C) The diluting segment of the tubules includes the ascending limb of the loop of Henle and about one-half of the convoluted portion of the loop of Henle is the major site for salt conservation. As the name implies, the function of the diluting segment is to dilute the tubular fluid. But really, the cells are specifically adapted for active transport of Cl^- ions from inside the tubular lumen into the peritubular fluid. This transport of negative chloride and positive sodium ions outward creates a net $+6$ mV charge inside the tubule, which causes Na^+ ions to diffuse out from lumen to peritubular fluid. This segment is also impermeable to water and more impermeable to urea. Hence, the remaining fluid is very dilute (except urea which is high). **(Ref. 2,** pp. 654–660)

384. (A) Normally all of the amino acids (as well as glucose) are not directly reabsorbed by active processes in the proximal tubule. They are co-transported with sodium ions. Specifically the electrochemical gradient for sodium entry provides the energy for glucose and amino acid transport across the brush border. **(Ref. 2,** p. 653)

385. (A) About 99% of the filtered Na^+ is reabsorbed by all the renal tubules. Approximately two-thirds of the filtered sodium is reabsorbed from the proximal tubule. The epithelial cells which line the proximal tubules have a "brush" border composed of very small microvilli. At the base of each cell are basal channels. The electrical potential within the cell is about -70 mV. Active transport of Na^+ occurs from inside the epithelial cell into the basal channels as well as into the spaces between the cells. This outward Na^+ transport reduces the Na^+ concentration inside, and because of the low concentration inside the cell there is a Na^+ concentration gradient between the cell and the tubular lumen fluid. As a result Na^+ will diffuse from the tubule through the brush border into the cell where it is actively carried into the peritubular fluid of the basal channels. So both the inside negative potential and the concentration gradient cause Na^+ to diffuse from the tubular lumen into the cell. This electrochemical gradient accounts for proximal Na^+ diffusion and amounts to about 65% of the filtered load. (**Ref. 2**, p. 663)

386. **(B)** The excretion of excess solutes and, hence, a concentrated urine is dependent on first creating a hyperosmolality of the medullary interstitial fluid. Normally, body fluid osmolality is 300 mOsm/L, while in the medullary tubules it approaches 1200 mOsm/L. In the thick ascending limb this active extrusion of Cl^- plus passive electrogenic absorption of Na^+ results in an increased medullary osmolality. These along with K^+ and C^{2+}, are carried downward into the inner medulla by the blood in the vasa recta. Ions are also transplanted from the collecting duct into the medullary interstitial fluid, mainly from active transport of Na^+ and electrogenic passive absorption of Cl^- along with the Na^+. In addition, when ADH concentration is high in the blood, large amounts of urea are also reabsorbed into the medullary fluid from the collecting duct. Finally, there is the passive transport of Na^+ and Cl^- into the inner medullary interstitium from the thin segment of the loop of Henle. This passive movement results from the high urea concentration in the medullary interstitium around the collecting ducts and promotes water osmosis out of the descending limb. As a result, there is a high NaCl concentration to twice normal inside the descending thin loop. Because of the high NaCl concentration, the ions move passively out of the thin segment and into the interstitium. All of these factors cause a marked increase in the medullary interstitial fluid and are referred to as the "countercurrent" fluid flow in the loop. As can be noted then, there may be occasions when the collecting duct has an equally high fluid

concentration as the loop, but it could be lower. The loop is always hyperosmotic. (**Ref. 2,** pp. 657–660)

387. (**C**)   The thick ascending section of the loop of Henle is the diluting segment of the tubule because of its high water impermeability. The cells of this area also are adapted specifically for active transport of Na^+ and Cl^- ions from inside the tubular lumen into the peritubular fluid. The low water permeability and active reabsorption of Na^+ and Cl^- means that in this area both the osmolality and NaCl concentration is lowered to levels below those in the surrounding fluid. (**Ref. 2,** pp. 657–660)

388. (**B**)   An increase in blood volume will result in a decrease in the secretion of renin from the juxtaglomerular apparatus. (**Ref. 2,** pp. 420–421)

389. (**B**)   Increased blood volume would decrease the presence of the angiotensin by decreasing the renin-assisted breakdown of globulin. (**Ref. 2,** pp. 670–671)

390. (**B**)   The adrenal cortex is stimulated by renin. Increased blood volume decreases renin release, hence, decreases adrenal cortical secretion. (**Ref. 2,** pp. 332–333)

391. (**B**)   The aldosterone secretion of the adrenal cortex is related to renin secretion and blood volume through a negative feedback relationship. (**Ref. 2,** pp. 332–333)

392. (**B**)   ADH secretion will be decreased by increased blood volume. This will allow the excretion of Na^+ and water to return blood volume toward normal. (**Ref. 2,** pp. 670–671)

393. (**B**)   The major function of ADH is to cause a decrease in urinary excretion of water (and Na^+) in order to return blood volume towards normal. (**Ref. 2,** p. 663)

394. (**A**)   Lower circulating levels of aldosterone will result in increased K^+ reabsorption. (**Ref. 1,** pp. 663, 665)

395. (**B**)   Water reabsorption will be inhibited by increased blood volume due to decreased secretion of ADH and aldosterone. (**Ref. 2,** pp. 654–660)

396. (B) The movement of fluid into the vascular system during the early stages of hemorrhagic shock causes the hematocrit to decrease. (**Ref. 2,** pp. 580–584)

397. (B) Decreased venous return will result in decreased cardiac output during shock. (**Ref. 2,** pp. 580–584)

398. (A) Peripheral resistance is increased during early stages of shock in an attempt to maintain normal blood pressure. (**Ref. 2,** pp. 580–584)

399. (A) Plasma protein concentration goes up during later stages of shock because of the release of protein from dying cells. (**Ref. 2,** pp. 580–584)

400. (B) The precapillary to post-capillary resistance ratio is decreased during irreversible shock. (**Ref. 2,** pp. 580–584)

401. (B) Mean arterial blood pressure is reduced during irreversible shock because the normal mechanisms for maintaining blood pressure are overwhelmed. (**Ref. 2,** pp. 580–584)

402. (E) Total body water makes up about 60% of the lean body weight. (**Ref. 2,** p. 670)

403. (B) Interstitial compartment water comprises approximately 15% of total lean body weight. (**Ref. 2,** p. 670)

404. (D) Intracellular water makes up approximately 40% of lean body weight. (**Ref. 2,** p. 670)

405. (A) Plasma water content comprises about 4% of lean body weight. (**Ref. 2,** p. 670)

406. (C) Extracellular fluid makes up about 20% of lean body weight. (**Ref. 2,** p. 670)

407. (A) Respiratory acidosis is caused by retention of CO_2 and may be produced by inhalation of gas mixture with high CO_2 content, voluntary breath holding, pulmonary insufficiency (as in emphysema), respiratory obstruction, respiratory center depression, or by paralysis of the respiratory muscles. The change in the blood is an increase in arterial hydrogen ion concentration and CO_2 tension. (**Ref. 2,** pp. 672–673)

408. (A) Because of the increased blood pCO_2 there will be an increase in HCO_3^- content during respiratory acidosis. The resulting renal excretion of chloride eventually will lead to an increase in buffer base. (**Ref. 2,** pp. 672–673)

409. (B) Respiratory alkalosis occurs when alveolar pCO_2 is lower than normal and results from an increase in alveolar ventilation. The effect on the blood is to decrease arterial hydrogen ion concentration and CO_2 tension. Causes of this condition include voluntary hyperventilation, anoxemia, hysteria, fever, dyspnea due to congestive heart failure, and lesions involving the brain stem. (**Ref. 2,** pp. 672–673)

410. (B) Following the lowered pCO_2 during respiratory alkalosis there will be a decrease in HCO_3^- content of the blood. The concomitant increase in plasma Cl^- concentration leads eventually to increased renal excretion of base, which lowers the buffer base content. (**Ref. 2,** pp. 672–673)

411. (B) Metabolic acidosis may be caused by an excess of fixed acid associated with metabolism, ingestion of acidifying salts, or by any condition in which more anions than cations are present in the circulation: The characteristic finding in metabolic acidosis is diminution in total base, decrease in buffer base, and an increase in arterial hydrogen ion content while CO_2 tension is reduced. (**Ref. 2,** pp. 672–673)

412. (B) As a result of the lower blood pCO_2 during metabolic acidosis, the HCO_3^- concentration will decrease. The condition is usually observed after massive diarrhea, particularly in infants. (**Ref. 2,** pp. 673–675)

413. (A) Metabolic alkalosis may occur either by a deficiency of fixed base (as following persistent vomiting) or by continuous loss of gastric juice. While the CO_2 content is raised following decreased ventilation, the total base and buffer base are decreased with an increase in plasma pH. The increase in blood pCO_2 follows the attempt by the lungs to restore the blood pH to normal. (**Ref. 2,** pp. 674–675)

414. **(A)** Following the increase in blood pCO_2 there will be an increase in plasma HCO_3^- during metabolic alkalosis. The arterial pH and HCO_3^- increase together, which enables metabolic alkalosis to be distinguished from respiratory alkalosis. (**Ref. 2,** pp. 674–675)

6

Cardiovascular Physiology

MULTIPLE CHOICE

DIRECTIONS (Questions 415–515): Each of the questions or incomplete statements below is followed by five suggested answers or completions. Select the **one** that is **best** in each case.

415. In cardiac muscle, sympathetic stimulation _____ developed tension, _____ +dT/dt and _____ −dT/dt
   A. increases, increases, increases
   B. decreases, decreases, decreases
   C. decreases, increases, increases
   D. increases, decreases, increases
   E. decreases, decreases, increases

416. The effect of increasing cycle length on the cardiac action potential of a follower cell is to
   A. decrease phase 2
   B. decrease phase 4
   C. increase the action potential duration
   D. decrease intracellular Ca^{2+} concentration
   E. C and D are correct

417. The following statements are correct regarding cardiac muscle **EXCEPT**
  A. no recruitment of fibers occurs, but it is present in skeletal muscle
  B. the cells are smaller (shorter) than skeletal muscle cells
  C. it shows treppe, which is the same as tetany seen in skeletal muscle
  D. passive tension is greater at L_{max} than in skeletal muscle
  E. there is no tone, like skeletal muscle, but unlike smooth muscle

418. Select the **INCORRECT** statement from the following
  A. spontaneous phase 4 depolarization is characteristic of a pacemaker cell in the heart
  B. cardiac muscle cells of the fast response type contain both fast and slow sodium ion channels
  C. the conduction through atrioventricular (AV) nodal cells is very slow compared with regular ventricular or atrial cells in the heart
  D. slow sodium ion channels can be blocked by tetrodotoxin
  E. Purkinje cells have a prolonged phase 2 depolarization

419. Second degree heart (AV) block
  A. always involves the progressive lengthening of the P-R interval until AV conduction fails, causing the loss of a ventricular depolarization
  B. is caused by a wandering atrial pacemaker
  C. usually involves retrograde conduction to atria
  D. always involves a lost ventricular depolarization every so many P waves
  E. most of the QRS complexes are wide and bizzare

420. Which of the following statements is **CORRECT**?
  A. In lead 1 the right arm is the positive electrode
  B. Repolarization of the ventricles occur from epicardium to endocardium (outside to inside)
  C. An inverted R wave is common in lead aVF
  D. The mean axis of the normal adult human heart is +150°
  E. The P wave results from depolarization of the right ventricle

421. Which one of the following frontal plane leads is matched with its **CORRECT** angle?
   A. II, −60°
   B. III, +120°
   C. aVF, −90°
   D. aVR, −30°
   E. aVL, +90°

422. Conduction of the wave of depolarization through the adult heart is slowest in the
   A. ventricle
   B. Purkinje fibers
   C. AV junctional tissue
   D. atrium
   E. ventricular endocardium

423. Which of the following statements regarding the cardiac cycle are **CORRECT**?
   A. The T wave begins immediately after the first heart sound
   B. The V wave of atrial/venous pulse occurs during and as the result of ventricular contraction
   C. Left atrial contraction slightly precedes right atrial contraction
   D. The third heart sound when heard occurs during atrial contraction
   E. Aortic flow is greatest during late ventricular ejection

424. Referring to Figure 16 of the cardiac cycle, C marks
   A. end-diastolic volume
   B. semilunar valve opening
   C. end-systolic volume
   D. isovolumic ventricular relaxation
   E. stroke volume

425. Referring to Figure 16 of the cardiac cycle, E marks
   A. AV valve opening
   B. isovolumic ventricular contraction
   C. isovolumic ventricular relaxation
   D. end-diastolic volume
   E. stroke work

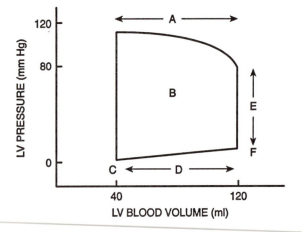

Figure 16 Left ventricle pressure-volume loop.

426. Regarding the heart sounds
   A. the aortic component of S2 normally occurs after the pulmonic component
   B. S3 is never heard in heart failure
   C. S1 results from mitral and tricuspid valve opening
   D. S4 results mainly from an abnormally robust left atrium
   E. the tricuspid component of S1 normally occurs before the mitral component

427. Which of the following statements is **INCORRECT**?
   A. Right atrial depolarization leads left atrial depolarization
   B. Left ventricular pressure remains above aortic pressure throughout ejection
   C. The pulmonic valve opens after the aortic valve
   D. The right ventricle begins to contract after the left ventricle
   E. The aortic valve closes before the pulmonic valve

428. During a cardiac catheterization the following data are collected from two 45-year-old men.

		Patient #1	Patient #2
Aorta:	Pressure (mm Hg)	140/50	95/65
	O_2 saturation (%)	95	96
Left ventricle:	Pressure (mm Hg)	140/15	95/9
	O_2 saturation (%)	95	96
Left atrium:	Pressure (mm Hg)	12	31
	O_2 saturation (%)	95	96
Pulmonary artery:	Pressure (mm Hg)	26/11	68/21
	O_2 saturation (%)	75	74
Right ventricle:	Pressure (mm Hg)	26/5	68/7
	O_2 saturation (%)	75	74
Right atrium:	Pressure (mm Hg)	5	6
	O_2 saturation (%)	75	74

Circle all the data in the preceding list for Patient #2 which are grossly abnormal and **select** the **one best** diagnosis for this individual from the following

A. mitral insufficiency
B. large ventricular septal defect
C. large atrial septal defect
D. systemic hypotension due to arteriovenous fistula (shunt)
E. tetralogy of Fallot

429. Regarding mitral valve motion
   A. the valve leaflets remain far apart throughout ventricular diastole
   B. papillary muscle contraction plays no role in valve closure
   C. the valve annulus area decreases during valve closure
   D. the posterior leaflet is the most mobile
   E. closure is entirely due to the increase in ventricular pressure

430. Which of the following statements regarding ventricular filling are **CORRECT?**
   A. Normally atrial contraction is responsible for 50% of ventricular filling at resting heart rate
   B. Inflow to the left ventricle is most rapid immediately after the opening of the mitral valve
   C. Expiration augments filling of the right ventricle
   D. A supine posture (lying down) inhibits filling of the right ventricle
   E. Early right ventricle filling is responsible for the C wave of the jugular venous pulse

431. Drugs that have a positive inotropic action on the heart
  A. increase the PEP (pre-ejection period)/LVET (left ventricular ejection time) ratio
  B. increase the ejection fraction
  C. both of the above are correct
  D. decrease left ventricular maximum dP/dt
  E. decrease left ventricular V_{max}

432. Cardiac hypertrophy in the adult human does all of the following **EXCEPT**
  A. serves to decrease wall stress (wall tension/unit wall thickness)
  B. comes about only through an increased size of pre-existing cardiac muscle cells
  C. when eccentric, involves mainly the laying down of new sarcomeres in series
  D. when concentric involves an increase in tension development during contraction
  E. is a pathological process always leading to ill health and eventual death

433. Movement upward along a normal Frank-Starling or ventricular function curve means the following **EXCEPT**
  A. increased performance is being achieved
  B. there is an increased inotropic state
  C. increased pre-loading has taken place
  D. could occur in the absence of neural innervation of the heart
  E. the muscle fiber have been stretched to a greater extent during diastole

434. In Figure 17,
  A. curve B expresses a decreased capability of the heart to serve as a pump
  B. curves A, B, and C are expressions of a relationship between fiber length and muscle tension
  C. curve C is an expression of cardiac capability that has been "improved" and is returning to "normal"
  D. curve A expresses a contractile capability of the heart that enables it to maximally respond to changes in venous return
  E. all are correct

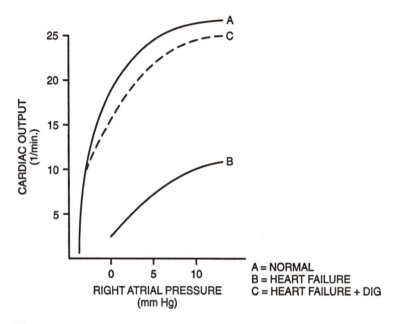

Figure 17 Three ventricular functional curves (A, B, C) representing the ability of the heart to function under various conditions.

435. A patient came to the cardiac catheterization laboratory and the following data were obtained for the left ventricle before and during medication

	Before	During
End-diastolic volume (ml)	120	110
End-systolic volume (ml)	40	40
End-diastolic pressure (mm Hg)	5.0	5.1
Mean ejection pressure (mm Hg)	75	95
End-diastolic radius (mm)	50	48
Mean ejection radius (mm)	40	40

If you assume that the ventricle was spherical throughout its cycle, you can conclude that the medication
A. increased the ventricle's afterload
B. increased the ventricle's preload
C. increased the ventricle's stroke volume
D. caused ventricular dilatation
E. decreased arterial blood pressure

436. Which of the following would **NOT** lead to increased diastolic stretching of the ventricle, thus increased performance during the subsequent contraction?
A. Assumption of the erect position
B. Increased venous tone (i.e., decreased wall compliance)
C. Inspiration
D. Increased blood volume
E. Increased atrial contraction

437. The shifting upward and to the left of a Frank-Starling or ventricular function curve may result from
A. increased ventricular pre-load
B. decreased heart rate
C. increased inotropicity and catecholamines
D. increased venous return to the heart
E. heart failure

438. Referring to Frank-Starling curves in Figure 18,
A. the line defined by D and C are at a higher inotropic state than the line defined by A and B
B. the line defined by A and B are at a higher inotropic state than the line defined by D and C
C. the pre-load at point C is greater than at point B
D. inotropicity at point C is greater than at point D
E. B and D are correct

439. Stimulation of cardiac adrenergic sympathetic neurons
A. increases the R-R interval of the ECG
B. decreases refractoriness at the AV node
C. decreases the rate of change of pressure in the left ventricle during isovolumetric contraction
D. decreases the stroke work of the ventricles
E. increases the end-systolic volume of the ventricles

440. In the resting subject, the greatest **NEGATIVE** arteriovenous oxygen (A-VO_2) concentration difference exists across the vascular bed of
A. kidney
B. lung
C. brain
D. heart
E. skeletal muscle

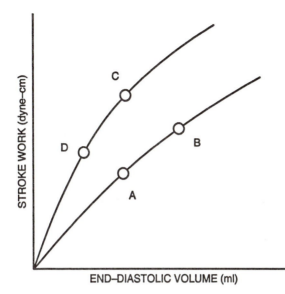

Figure 18 Ventricular function or Frank-Starling curves for the heart.

441. The following data were obtained from a patient before and during medication

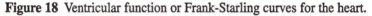

	Before	During
Oxygen concentration (ml of O_2/ml blood)		
Right femoral artery	.190	.190
Right femoral vein	.120	.140
Pulmonary artery	.130	.135
Coronary sinus	.06	.04
Oxygen consumption of patient (ml O_2/min)	250	260
End-diastolic volume of left ventricle (ml)	150	160
Mean ejection pressure of left ventricle (mm Hg)	90	100
Aortic pressure (mm Hg)	120/80	115/85
Heart rate (cycles/min)	75	100

What conclusions can you draw from these data? The medication

A. increased the arteriovenous oxygen (A-V$_{O_2}$) concentration difference across the right thigh
B. increased the arteriovenous oxygen (A-V$_{O_2}$) concentration difference across the coronary vessels
C. did both A and B
D. decreased left ventricular pre-load
E. decreased left ventricular pre-load and minute work

442. The following data are collected from a patient

Body weight	65 kg
Respiratory tidal volume	230 ml
O_2 consumption	150 ml/min
Heart rate	75/min
Femoral artery O_2 concentration	20 ml/dl (pO_2 = 100 mm Hg)
Femoral vein O_2 concentration	12 ml/dl (pO_2 = 35 mm Hg)
Pulmonary artery O_2 concentration	14 ml/dl (pO_2 = 40 mm Hg)

What is the cardiac output of this patient?
A. Less than 1600 ml/min
B. Between 1600 and 2000 ml/min
C. Between 2050 and 2400 ml/min
D. Between 2450 and 2800 ml/min
E. More than 2800 ml/min

443. All of the following are correct regarding oxygen utilization **EXCEPT**
A. may be increased by the myocardium by increasing blood flow rate
B. is always less than oxygen delivery
C. may be increased greatly by the myocardium by increasing oxygen extraction
D. is increased by an increased myocardial inotropic state or movement up a ventricular function curve
E. is equal to the product of blood flow rate and arteriovenous oxygen (A-V_{O_2}) difference

444. Referring to Figure 19,
A. A represents venous blood oxygen content
B. E represents arterial blood oxygen content
C. F represents arteriovenous oxygen (A-V_{O_2}) difference
D. D is myocardium
E. B is kidney

445. The effects of endurance exercise training are the following **EXCEPT**
A. increased maximal heart rate
B. increased skeletal muscle capillary density

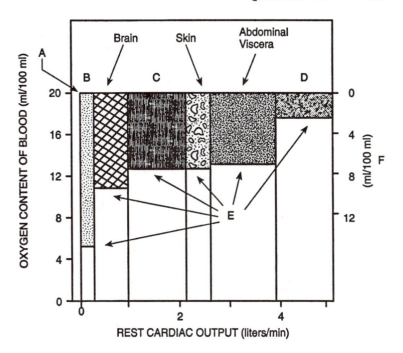

Figure 19 Arterial and venous blood oxygen contents, arteriovenous oxygen differences, and blood flow rates of various organs and tissues in the body.

    C. increased central blood volume
    D. increased maximal cardiac output
    E. increased skeletal muscle oxidative enzymes

446. An individual standing quietly begins to run. His oxygen consumption increases eightfold. What other changes occur in response to the exercise **EXCEPT?**
    A. A decrease in cardiac parasympathetic tone
    B. An increase in left ventricle end-systolic volume
    C. A shift of the Frank-Starling (ventricular function) curve to the left
    D. An increase in the mean systemic arteriovenous oxygen (A-V$_{O_2}$) difference
    E. An increase in ventricular positive and negative dP/dt coupled to an increase in heart rate

447. The following are correct regarding circulation time **EXCEPT**
   A. it is more than 10 minutes through the splenic circulation while at rest
   B. it is more dependent on what happens in the arteries than in the veins
   C. it is decreased generally by exercise
   D. it is longest through the veins, venous sinuses, and spleen
   E. it is the average time taken for an erythrocyte, or any particle in the blood, to move from one point in the circulation to another point

448. The following data were obtained from a patient before and during medication

	Before	During
Oxygen concentration (ml of O_2/ml blood)		
Right femoral artery	.190	.190
Right femoral vein	.120	.140
Pulmonary artery	.130	.135
Coronary sinus	.06	.04
Oxygen consumption of patient (ml O_2/min)	250	260
End-diastolic volume of left ventricle (ml)	150	160
Mean ejection pressure of left ventricle (mm Hg)	90	100
Aortic pressure (mm Hg)	120/80	115/85
Heart rate (cycles/min)	75	100

What conclusions can you draw from these data? The medication
   A. increased the arteriovenous oxygen (A-V$_{O2}$) concentration difference across the right thigh
   B. increased the arteriovenous oxygen (A-V$_{O2}$) concentration difference across the coronary vessels
   C. did both A and B
   D. decreased left ventricular pre-load
   E. decreased left ventricular afterload

449. Referring to Figure 20 illustrating cardiovascular reserve
   A. F represents cardiovascular reserve
   B. D represents residual volume
   C. B minus A represents arteriovenous oxygen (A-V$_{O2}$) difference at a high work rate

CARDIOVASCULAR RESERVE

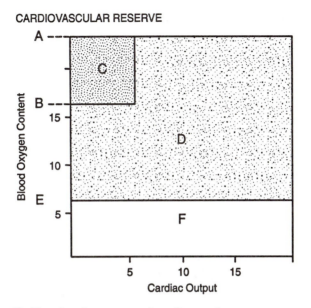

Figure 20 Showing the concept of cardiovascular reserve.

    D. E is venous oxygen content at a high work rate
    E. A and C are correct

450. Coronary blood flow
    A. is greatest during diastole in the left ventricle
    B. may increase twelvefold at maximal myocardial work levels
    C. is dependent upon the difference between aortic pressure and coronary sinus pressure
    D. is not affected by heart rate or myocardial contractile state
    E. is increased by incomplete ventricular relaxation

451. Which of the following is the most common cause of an increased coronary blood flow?
    A. A decreased coronary perfusion pressure
    B. An increased ventricular diastolic pressure
    C. An increased stimulation of alpha-adrenergic receptors in the heart
    D. An increased stimulation of beta-1 adrenergic receptors in the heart
    E. An increased stimulation of beta-2 adrenergic receptors in the heart

452. Which of the following is NOT an indication of coronary ischemia?

    A. A higher lactate concentration in the coronary sinus than in a coronary artery

    B. Release of enzyme (LDH, CPK) into the coronary venous blood

    C. An acute alteration in height of the ST segment

    D. A decreased coronary arteriovenous oxygen concentration difference

    E. An acute change in the T wave

453. Referring to a pressure-flow curve for the coronary circulation in Figure 21,

    A. A represents an autoregulatory region

    B. B represents an area of maximal vasodilation

    C. C is outside the autoregulatory region

    D. E represents an area of maximal vasodilation

    E. D represents an area of minimal vasoconstriction

Figure 21 Illustrating the concept of autoregulation of blood flow.

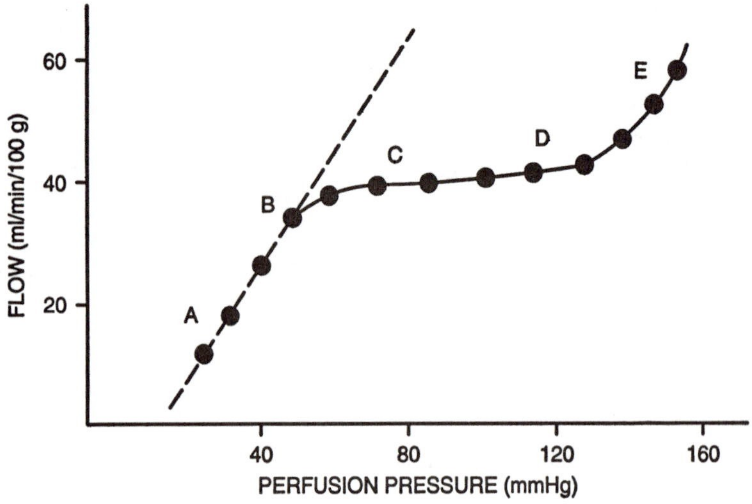

454. Of the following, which blood vessel carries blood of the highest oxygen content in the fetus?
   A. Ductus arteriosus
   B. Descending aorta
   C. Umbilical veins
   D. Pulmonary vein
   E. Thoracic inferior vena cava

455. Different animals have different approaches for delivering oxygen to the fetus. With regard to the variety of strategies
   A. the oxygen dissociation curve (ODC) of the blood of the fetal lamb is left-shifted some 17 mm Hg compared to the mother's blood
   B. the situation in humans for the relative positions of the ODCs in fetus versus mother is similar to that of sheep
   C. increasing fetal blood acidosis acts to increase the difference between the positions of the ODCs of the fetus and the mother
   D. increasing maternal alkalosis acts to increase the difference between the positions of the ODCs of the fetus and the mother
   E. the p50 value of the normal human is approximately 36 mm Hg

456. Hypoxia has the following effects on the fetus **EXCEPT**
   A. increase in plasma catecholamines
   B. increase in use of glycolytic pathway and lactate
   C. increase in heart rate
   D. decrease on fetal blood pH
   E. decrease in fetal oxygen consumption

457. You are a pediatric cardiologist and do oximetry (measurement of blood oxygen concentration) on a young patient with suspected congenital heart disease. There is no evidence of cyanosis. The following results are obtained

Site	Oxygen saturation (%)
Inferior vena cava	69
Right atrium	68
Right ventricle	83
Pulmonary artery	83
Left atrium	98
Left ventricle	98
Aorta	98

The values above are most consistent with

A. atrial septal defect
B. tetralogy of Fallot
C. ventricular septal defect
D. patent ductus arteriosus
E. isolated pulmonic stenosis

458. At birth
A. the foramen ovale will only close if the umbilical cord is clamped
B. right to left shunting of blood through the ductus arteriosus continues until the ductus closes
C. a transitional or neonatal circulation is usually seen for some time after birth
D. pulmonary vascular resistance falls shortly before birth because of pressure in the birth canal
E. all are correct

459. Resistance to blood flow
A. is directly determinable based on measurements of blood pressure alone
B. of several resistances in series is equal to the sum of the reciprocals of each of the individual resistances
C. is usually expressed ohms
D. of the large veins, usually represents less than 10% of total systemic peripheral resistance
E. of the pulmonary circulation, is about equivalent to that of the systemic circulation

460. The Poiseuille equation applies exactly only to fluid systems involving
   A. fluids whose viscosity is dependent on shear rate
   B. distensible conduits
   C. laminar flow
   D. fluids whose viscosity is dependent on conduit caliber
   E. A and C are correct

461. In Figure 22 which of the following hemodynamic situation(s) exist(s)?
   A. The blood flow profile is turbulent in nature
   B. The greatest pressure in this vessel exists at the vessel walls
   C. The least number of RBCs will flow in lamina A
   D. Streamline A is moving faster than streamline B, C, or D
   E. B and D are correct

462. Perfusion pressure
   A. is equal to transmural pressure
   B. of the systemic circulation is usually equal to or slightly less than the mean arterial pressure
   C. of the coronary circulation is uninfluenced by ventricular luminal pressure
   D. is the only part of total fluid energy which influences blood flow
   E. from arterial to venous vessels is greater in the feet than in the brain because of gravity

Figure 22 Blood flow in a large artery such as the aorta.

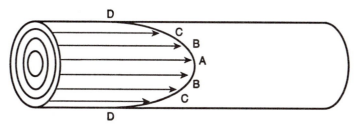

AORTIC BLOOD FLOW

463. A patient responded to a drug with a decrease in her total systemic peripheral resistance and an increase in mean arterial pressure. Which of the following best characterizes the mode of action of the drug? It probably produced
  A. a vasoconstriction and an increase in cardiac output
  B. a vasoconstriction and a decrease in cardiac output
  C. a vasodilation and an increase in cardiac output
  D. a vasodilation and a decrease in cardiac output
  E. a decrease in venous return of blood to the heart

464. The Fahraeus effect
  A. results in a rise in blood viscosity in blood vessels smaller than 1 mm radius
  B. occurs with Newtonian fluids
  C. results only as the result of axial flow of red blood cells
  D. involves a fall in dynamic hematocrit in small vessels
  E. is due mainly to red blood cell orientational changes as blood begins to move

465. Regarding a non-Newtonian fluid such as blood, which of the following is **CORRECT**
  A. the cell-free or slippage layer is larger in capillaries than in arterioles
  B. viscosity increases in non-capillary vessels of radius less than 1 mm
  C. dynamic hematocrit decreases in blood vessels down to 10–15 μm
  D. viscosity increases with increasing flow velocity
  E. erythrocyte and plasma velocity are identical in large and small blood vessels

466. The following are correct regarding total fluid energy of the blood (per mL) **EXCEPT**
  A. it is made up of a large fractional contribution by kinetic energy relative to pressure energy in the vena cavae
  B. it is primarily dissipated against gavitational forces
  C. it is the sum of pressure, kinetic, and gravitational potential energies
  D. it is much greater in the aorta than in the vena cavae
  E. it is not represented in the Poiseuille equation

467. The following are correct regarding the Poiseuille equation **EXCEPT**
   A. flow will increase when viscosity decrease
   B. flow is inversely proportional to vessel length
   C. flow is directly proportional to radius to the fourth power
   D. physiologically, perfusion pressure is the most important factor in determining flow
   E. turbulence and distensible tubes do not compromise the use of the equation

468. In the normal hemodynamic situation (see Figure 23), which of the following relationships operate
   A. P_T, exerted on the wall, is the difference between P_i and P_E
   B. the relationship between pressure and wall tension is largely determined by vessel radius and may be expressed as $T = PR$
   C. A and B are correct
   D. P_I exerted on the wall is independent of P_E
   E. all are correct

Figure 23 The forces (arrows) acting on a blood vessel: (P_I intravascular pressure; (P_E extravascular pressure; (T) circumferential tension in the vessel wall.

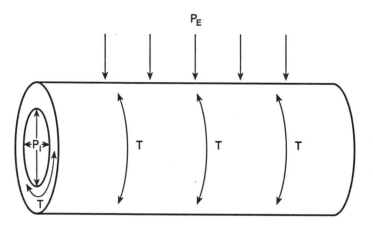

469. The largest fractional volume of blood in the circulation is normally contained in
  A. veins
  B. vena cavae
  C. capillaries
  D. arterioles
  E. aorta

470. The greatest single source of resistance to blood flow in the systemic circulation is encountered in the
  A. aorta
  B. vena cavae
  C. arterioles
  D. capillaries
  E. terminal veins

471. The Windkessel effect has the greatest influence on magnitude of the pulse pressure in the
  A. aorta
  B. capillaries
  C. venules
  D. veins
  E. arterioles

472. Total resistance of a number of resistances in series in a vascular system is equal to
  A. the sum of the reciprocals of each individual resistance
  B. the product of each individual resistance
  C. the sum of each individual resistance
  D. the product of the reciprocals of each individual resistance
  E. the value of the largest individual resistance

473. Decreased venous wall compliance may result from the following EXCEPT
  A. increased blood-borne epinephrine producing smooth muscle contraction
  B. increased hydrostatic pressure resulting from change of posture
  C. bed rest, space flight, and alcohol imbibition
  D. norepinephrine release from nerves innervating vascular smooth muscle
  E. increased vessel wall collagen content

474. During aging in man, the following usually occur **EXCEPT**
  A. maximum heart rate decreases
  B. pulse wave velocity in arteries increases
  C. pulse pressure decreases
  D. systolic arterial blood pressure increases
  E. blood vessel wall compliance decreases

475. The law of LaPlace states that wall tension of a blood vessel is related to
  A. the sum of pressure and radius
  B. the product of pressure and radius
  C. the ratio of pressure to radius
  D. the product of pressure and vessel length
  E. radius alone

476. Critical closure pressure
  A. is independent of the state of vascular smooth muscle contraction
  B. is the perfusion pressure at and below which vessel closure occurs and flow becomes zero
  C. remains constant over time for a particular organ or tissue
  D. is not influenced by autonomic sympathetic outflow
  E. B and C are correct

477. The stimulation of alpha-adrenergic receptors causes
  A. an increased heart rate
  B. cutaneous vasodilation
  C. skeletal muscle vasoconstriction
  D. A and B are correct
  E. B and C are correct

478. Angiotensin II has the following effects **EXCEPT**
  A. stimulates antidiuretic hormone release
  B. stimulates renin release
  C. stimulates thirst
  D. is a powerful vasoconstrictor
  E. stimulates aldosterone release

479. In the absence of cardiovascular reflexes (receptors and nervous system)
   A. a decrease in heart rate increases pulse pressure
   B. an increase in stroke volume decreases pulse pressure
   C. a decrease in compliance decreases pulse pressure
   D. an increase in resistance increases pulse pressure
   E. neither heart rate, stroke volume, compliance, nor resistance have any effect on pulse pressure

480. Depression of the central nervous system prevents an intravenous injection of norepinephrine from causing
   A. a decreased heart rate
   B. an increased heart rate
   C. an increased heart rate and cardiac output
   D. vasodilation
   E. an increase in arterial blood pressure

481. The carotid sinus baroreceptors
   A. are small bean-like structures located near the bifurcation of the common carotid artery
   B. respond to increased arterial blood pressure by an increased rate of nerve firing
   C. are more sensitive to falling than to constant or rising arterial blood pressure
   D. are less sensitive than the aortic baroreceptors to arterial blood pressure
   E. serve to decrease cardiac parasympathetic tone when resting blood pressure rises above the set point

482. Central blood volume is
   A. decreased by the weightlessness of space flight
   B. increased by blood transfusion
   C. increased by standing upright from lying down
   D. increased by positive pressure breathing
   E. unaffected by the Valsalva maneuver

483. Regarding changes in the maternal circulation during gestation, which of the following is **CORRECT**?
   A. Blood volume remains constant during gestation
   B. Plasma volume increases during gestation
   C. Uterine blood flow increases twofold or less

D. Cardiac output increases through increases in heart rate alone

E. Diphosphoglycerate is depressed in maternal blood due to hypoventilation

484. An increase in the osmolality of the extracellular compartment associated with a reduction in volume will

A. stimulate the volume and osmoreceptors, decreasing ADH secretion

B. inhibit the volume and osmoreceptors, increasing ADH secretion

C. inhibit the volume and osmoreceptors, decreasing ADH secretion

D. inhibit the volume and stimulate the osmoreceptors, increasing ADH secretion

E. none of the above

485. The following values were recorded in an experiment

capillary hydrostatic pressure = 25 mm Hg
capillary oncotic pressure = 30 mm Hg
tissue hydrostatic pressure = 3 mm Hg
tissue oncotic pressure = 10 mm Hg

The net forces favor

A. filtration by 2 mm Hg

B. reabsorption by 2 mm Hg

C. filtration by 12 mm Hg

D. reabsorption by 12 mm Hg

E. filtration by 42 mm Hg

486. The names Adolph Fick and Otto Loewi are associated, respectively, with discoveries of

A. cholinergic influences and methods of cardiac output estimation

B. methods of cardiac output estimation and cholinergic influences

C. the Hg sphygmomanometer and the kymograph

D. the kymograph and the Hg sphygmomanometer

E. the vasomotor reflexes and blood pressure measurement

487. Marey's law states that
   A. blood pressure and heart rate bear a direct relationship
   B. blood pressure determines glomerular filtration rate
   C. blood pressure and heart rate bear a reciprocal relationship
   D. heart rate is determined by the sinus rhythm
   E. heart rate and blood pressure are unrelated

488. The following are **CORRECT** regarding the Valsalva maneuver **EXCEPT**
   A. may be dangerous in individuals with coronary heart disease
   B. produces increased heart rate during stage 1
   C. decreases venous return to the heart
   D. results in decreased arterial blood pressure in stages 2 and 3, which may produce syncope
   E. is commonly used by normal individuals

489. Which of the following statements is **INCORRECT** regarding the diving reflex?
   A. It results from increased pCO_2 and depressed pH and pO_2 acting on the peripheral chemoreceptors
   B. It is manifested by reflex bradycardia
   C. It is exacerbated by increased water (hydrostatic) pressure during a dive
   D. It is manifested in man by an increased systemic peripheral resistance and arterial blood pressure
   E. It is due to increased vagal parasympathetic tone to the heart and increased sympathetic outflow to systemic arteries and arterioles

490. Development of orthostatic hypotension would be least likely to develop following
   A. long-continued bedrest
   B. standing immobile in heat
   C. alcohol consumption
   D. endurance exercise
   E. denervation of the carotid and aortic baroreceptors

491. Which of the following statements is **CORRECT**?
   A. Heart rate rises and blood pressure falls during stage II of the Valsalva maneuver
   B. Hyperventilation produces dizziness because too much oxygen reaches the brain

C. During orthostasis, central blood volume decreases, arterial blood pressure falls, and heart increases reflexly
D. A and C are correct
E. None are correct

492. In inspiratory tachycardia in the human
 A. left ventricular pre-load increases and consequently stroke volume rises
 B. "spill-over" occurs from the respiratory center to the cardio-vascular center, accelerating heart rate
 C. venous return to the right heart and pulmonary vascular volume decrease
 D. right ventricular pre-load declines and consequently stroke volume decreases
 E. heart rate and systemic arterial blood pressure increase

493. Bleeding time
 A. measures the rate of bleeding from a large puncture
 B. is normally about 2 to 3 min
 C. is significantly longer in hemophilia
 D. is independent of platelet concentration
 E. is normally about 6 to 8 min

494. Latent pacemaker activity in the heart resides in the
 A. left ventricular muscle
 B. bundle of His
 C. N layer of the AV node
 D. the Purkinje network
 E. left atrial muscle

495. It is impossible to tetanize a heart because
 A. there is a long mechanical refractory period
 B. the electrical refractory period and the mechanical contractile response are of almost equivalent duration
 C. the mechanical contractile event is usually shorter than the duration of the electrical depolarization
 D. the Ca^{2+} transport mechanism in heart muscle is responsible for the prolonged refractoriness
 E. heart muscles do not contain Ca^{2+}

496. During the reduced ejection phase of the left ventricle, which one of the following is true?
   A. Left atrial pressure is falling
   B. Aortic flow velocity is rapidly decreasing
   C. Aortic pressure is falling below left ventricular pressure
   D. Left ventricular pressure is constant
   E. The tricuspid valves are closed

497. Both cyanosis and systemic arterial blood hypoxemia may occur in the presence of
   A. potassium cyanide (KCN) poisoning
   B. a low cardiac output
   C. regions of abnormally low ventilation/perfusion (V/Q) ratio
   D. some regions of the lung being relatively more perfused than others
   E. heart rates between 40 and 50 beats/min

498. Pressure in the main pulmonary artery
   A. will approximately double if cardiac output doubles
   B. will approximately double if one lung is removed
   C. is lowered by a local vasodilator effect of alveolar hypoxia
   D. is always high enough to perfuse the uppermost parts of a human lung
   E. is not inversely proportional to cardiac output

499. Cardiac work is most nearly equal to the
   A. area of the pressure–volume diagram
   B. tension–time index
   C. kinetic energy imparted to movement of blood
   D. systolic blood pressure
   E. heart rate

500. Sympathetic adrenergic stimulation results in
   A. vasoconstriction in all tissues
   B. increased coronary blood flow
   C. increased muscle blood flow
   D. increased skin blood flow
   E. vasodilation in all tissues

501. According to the myogenic theory of autoregulation of blood flow, increasing arteriolar blood pressure leads to
   A. an elevation of tissue blood flow
   B. a decreased vascular resistance
   C. an increased vascular resistance
   D. decreased vascular tone
   E. decreased blood flow

502. The most important factor in improving the ability of the heart to increase blood flow to peripheral tissue in exercise is
   A. increased oxygen extraction from the blood by the heart
   B. increased myocardial efficiency independent of oxygen needs of the organ
   C. increased coronary blood flow
   D. increased venomotor tone
   E. decreased circulating catecholamines

503. According to the Poiseuille relationship, doubling vessel length should cause blood flow to
   A. double
   B. halve
   C. increase 16 times
   D. decrease
   E. not change since there is no relationship between length and blood flow

504. The length–tension relationship in cardiac muscle allows the heart to make automatic adjustments in its output. This is accomplished by
   A. a decrease in the potential force of contraction as the resting (diastolic) fiber length is increased (over a normal physiologic range)
   B. an increase in the amount and rate of shortening following an increase in resting (diastolic) fiber length (over a normal physiologic range)
   C. a reduction in the contractility of the heart muscle following an increased diastolic filling
   D. a change in the amount of actin and myosin per fiber
   E. alterations in the Ca^{2+} uptake by the sarcoplasmic reticulum

505. The calcified, rigid aorta often seen in elderly people requires an increased cardiac performance for an adequate cardiac output because it
   A. has a smaller than normal diameter and so increases the resistance to outflow from the heart
   B. accommodates less blood than normal between 90 and 150 mm Hg pressure and so requires a higher than normal ejection pressure
   C. gives less elastic recoil during diastole and so reduces the load and thus the contribution of homeometric autoregulation
   D. tends to prevent movement of the base of the heart and so reduces effective venous return
   E. decreases the amount of calcium available to the cardiac muscle

506. An adult male is seen in the clinic with the following findings

Cardiac output	5 L/min
Systolic pressure	200 mm Hg
Diastolic pressure	120 mm Hg
Heart rate	80 bpm
Plasma catecholamines	normal
Blood volume	5 L
Total peripheral resistance	increased
Plasma angiotensin	normal

From the above data, it should be concluded that the patient is
   A. hypertensive due to excessive cardiac activity
   B. suffering from essential hypertension
   C. in hypotension of renal origin
   D. hypertensive as a result of excessive adrenomedullary secretion
   E. suffering from hypertension of neural origin

507. Which of the following factors would be expected to contribute to the peripheral edema commonly observed in congestive heart failure?
   A. Decreased arterial pressure, increased serum sodium, increased tissue hydrostatic pressure
   B. Decreased arterial pressure, decreased venous pressure, increased hematocrit

C. Increased venous pressure, decreased serum proteins, increased plasma volume
D. Decreased arterial pH, increased skeletal muscle activity, increased sympathetic tone
E. Decreased blood volume, decreased aldosterone secretion, decreased venous pressure

508. During stress or exercise, which of the following cardiovascular system reserves have the largest potential for increasing oxygen supply to the tissues?
A. Increased blood arterial oxygen content
B. Increased blood flow resulting from increased stroke volume
C. Increased extraction of oxygen from the blood
D. Increased arterial blood pressure
E. Increased venous blood pressure

MATCHING

DIRECTIONS: For the next four questions (509–512) **select answers** from the **two lists.**

Questions 509 and 510:

A. aorta
B. capillary
C. pulmonary artery
D. pulmonary vein
E. left atrium
F. left ventricle
G. pre-capillary sphincter
H. right atrium
I. right coronary artery
J. right ventricle
K. systemic arteriole
L. systemic artery
M. vein
N. venule

For each **structure** listed, select the **one most likely** to answer the following questions.

509. What site in the circulation shows the greatest Windkessel effect (i.e., hydraulic filtering)?

510. Using an indwelling catheter, a blood sample and blood pressure measurements are made on a normal patient, giving values of 73% saturation and 28/15 mm Hg, respectively. At what point in the circulation is the catheter tip drawing the samples/making the measurements?

Questions 511 and 512:

    A. orthostasis
    B. exercise
    C. congestive heart failure
    D. inspiratory tachycardia
    E. hyperventilation
    F. syncope
    G. valsalva maneuver
    H. Muller maneuver
    I. diving reflex

For each **statement** listed, select the **one most likely** to answer the following questions.

511. Condition characterized by simultaneous bradycardia and falling arterial blood pressure.

512. During stage II, heart rate rises reflexly as arterial blood pressure decreases.

DIRECTIONS (Questions 513–515): This section consists of a situation followed by a series of questions. Study the **situation** and select the **one best answer** to each question.

Questions 513–515: The following data were obtained from two patients

	Patient A	Patient B
Cardiac output (CO)	—	—
Mean blood pressure	—	—
Heart rate	100	150
O_2 consumption (mL/min)	250	—
Venous O_2 (mL/100 mL)	14.5	—
Arterial O_2 (mL/100 mL)	19.0	—
Stroke volume (mL/beat)	—	70

513. The cardiac output in patient A is (in L/min)
   A. 3.0 L/min
   B. 5.5 L/min
   C. 7.5 L/min
   D. 12.0 L/min
   E. 20.0 L/min

514. The stroke volume in patient A is (in mL/beat)
   A. 55 mL/beat
   B. 70 mL/beat
   C. 80 mL/beat
   D. 100 mL/beat
   E. 150 mL/beat

515. The CO in patient B is (in L/min)
   A. 3.0 L/min
   B. 5.5 L/min
   C. 7.0 L/min
   D. 8.0 L/min
   E. 10.5 L/min

DIRECTIONS (Questions 516–547): Each group of questions below consists of a set of lettered components, followed by a list of numbered words or phrases. For each numbered word or phrase, select the **one** lettered component that is **most closely** associated with it. Each lettered component may be selected once, more than once, or not at all.

Questions 516 and 517 (Figure 24):

    A. curve A
    B. curve B

516. The cardiac output of the right ventricle is represented by

517. The cardiac output of the left ventricle is represented by

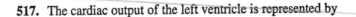

Figure 24 Relationship between cardiac output and end-diastolic pressure (mm Hg).

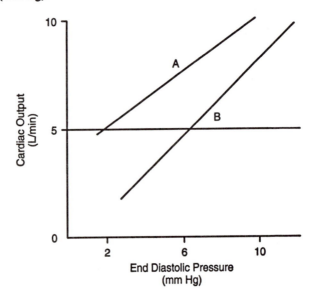

Questions 518–520 (Figure 25):

    A. site A
    B. site B
    C. site C
    D. site D
    E. site E

518. Major vascular resistance is

519. Major fluid exchange is

520. Lowest erythrocyte linear velocity is

Figure 25 Changes in mean systemic blood pressure as the blood goes from the aorta through the various vessel types.

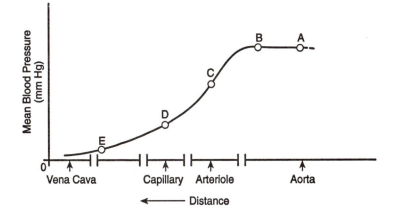

Questions 521–526:

    A. first event
    B. second event
    C. third event
    D. fourth event
    E. fifth event
    F. sixth event

Starting from the P wave, indicate the order in which the following events occur

521. AV valve opens

522. Aortic valve closes

523. Q wave

524. T wave

525. AV valve closes

526. Aortic valve opens

Questions 527–531:

    A. first heart sound
    B. second heart sound
    C. P wave
    D. Q wave
    E. T wave

527. Period of isovolumetric contraction

528. Immediately precedes isovolumic contraction

529. Occurs during ventricular ejection phase

530. Immediately precedes atrial contraction

531. Period of isometric relaxation

Questions 532–537:

    A. increases from normal average value
    B. decreases from the normal average value
    C. does not change from the normal average value

532. Mean arterial pressure in a patient with mitral stenosis

533. Left atrial pressure in a patient with aortic regurgitation

534. Cardiac output in a mitral stenotic patient

535. Left ventricular volume in a patient with mitral stenosis

536. Left atrial volume in a patient with mitral stenosis

537. Total blood volume in a patient with aortic regurgitation

Questions 538–547 (Figure 26):

    A. P wave
    B. U wave
    C. T wave
    D. QRS complex
    E. PR interval
    F. ST segment
    G. QT interval
    H. Q wave
    I. S wave
    J. R wave

538. Deflection #1

539. Deflection #2

540. Deflection #3

541. Deflection #4

542. Deflection #5

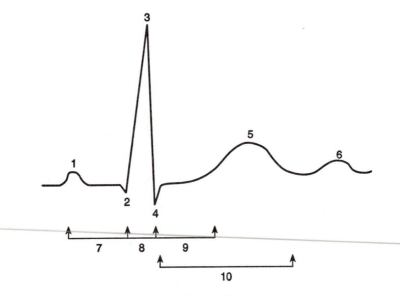

Figure 26

543. Deflection #6

544. Period #7

545. Period #8

546. Period #9

547. Period #10

Cardiovascular Physiology

Answers and Discussion

415. (A) Sympathetic stimulation of cardiac muscle increases developed tension, +dT/dt and −dT/dt by increasing inotropic state. **(Ref. 1,** pp. 404–405)

416. (E) Increasing cycle length increases the duration of the action potential and decreases intracellular Ca^{2+} concentration. It also increases the duration of phases 2 and 4 of the action potential. **(Ref. 1,** pp. 379–380)

417. (C) Treppe is not the same as tetany in skeletal muscle; in that, treppe consists of discrete twitches where complete or nearly complete relaxation occurs before the next begins, while in tetany, individual twitches merge into one continuous contraction. **(Ref. 1,** pp. 397–399)

418. (D) Tetrodotoxin only blocks the fast sodium channels. **(Ref. 1,** p. 374)

419. (D) In the Mobitz II type of second degree heart block, P-R interval remains constant prior to loss of ventricular depolarization. Second degree heart block usually involves the sinus node and orthograde conduction. As a consequence the QRS complexes are generally normal in shape. **(Ref. 1,** pp. 390–391)

420. **(B)** Repolarization of the ventricles occurs in the opposite direction from depolarization (i.e., endocardium to epicardium). In lead I the positive electrode is at the left arm. By definition the R wave is always upright. The mean electrical axis of the heart is approximately +60°. The P wave results from depolarization of the atria. (**Ref. 1,** pp. 388–389)

421. **(B)** Lead III is a bipolar limb lead with the positive electrode attached to the left leg. Its angle in the frontal plane is +120°. The other leads and their angles are: lead II, +60°; lead aVF, +90°; lead aVR, −150°; lead aVL, −30°. (**Ref. 1,** pp. 388–389)

422. **(C)** Conduction velocity through the AV junctional tissue and the AV node is approximately .05 m/sec; whereas, velocity is .3–2.0 m/sec in the bundle branches, Purkinje fibers and ventricular myocardium. (**Ref. 1,** pp. 382–383)

423. **(B)** The T wave occurs well after the first heart sound and ends just before the second heart sound. Right atrial contraction leads left atrial contraction, since the sinus node resides in the wall of the right atrium and the wave of depolarization spreads through the right side first. The third heart sound, when heard, occurs during the rapid filling phase of the cardiac cycle. Aortic flow is greatest just after the aortic valve opens and declines rapidly during later ejection. (**Ref. 1,** pp. 407–408)

424. **(C)** End-sytolic volume. (**Ref. 1,** pp. 411–412)

425. **(B)** Isovolumic ventricular contraction. (**Ref. 1,** pp. 411–412)

426. **(D)** The first heart sound results mainly from AV valve closure, and the second heart sound from semilunar valve closure. Because the left ventricle begins contracting a short time before the right ventricle, the mitral component of S_1 precedes the tricuspid component. Because of greater aortic and pulmonic afterload, the aortic component of S_2 precedes the pulmonic component. S_3 is very often heard in heart failure and results from abnormal rapid filling. S_4 is produced by an abnormally robust left atrium, as following chronic mitral regurgitation. (**Ref. 1,** pp. 409–410)

427. **(C)** Because pulmonary artery pressure is only a fraction of aortic pressure, the right ventricle need raise its pressure only a frac-

tion of the left ventricle in order for the semi-lunar valve to open. Since the two ventricles contract almost simultaneously, the valve opening pressure is achieved earlier by the right ventricle. (**Ref. 2,** pp. 515–516)

428. (**A**) The systolic pressures for the aorta and left ventricle are low, while left atrial pressure is elevated. Pulmonary artery and right ventricle pressures are also elevated. Leakage through the mitral valve ventricular systole lowers left ventricle pressure and raises it in the left atrium, and also elevates pressure upstream in a backwardly directed fashion. There is no "oxygen step-up" in right atrium or right ventricle, so septal defect in either is not indicated. Arteriovenous fistula is unlikely since the mixed-venous oxygen saturation is normal (i.e., 74%). Lack of significant cyanosis rules out tetralogy of Fallot. (**Ref. 1,** pp. 410–411)

429. (**C**) The mitral valve, has 2 cusps, or leaflets, attached through the chordae tendineae to papillary muscles embedded in the wall of the left ventricle. The anterior leaflet is most mobile. Valve closure is complex, involving eddy currents resulting from atrial contraction, papillary muscle contraction, and the sphinteric action of the valve annulus. Closure is not solely or even mainly due to rising ventricular pressure! Papillary muscle contraction also prevents valve eversion into the atrium which would cause regurgitation. Valve opening involves an initial opening during rapid filling, partial closure during diastasis, re-opening during atrial systole, and a final closure immediately prior to ventricular systole. This is the typical M pattern seen with echocardiography. (**Ref. 1,** pp. 407–408)

430. (**B**) At rest, atrial contraction contributes approximately 15% to ventricular filling. Ventricular filling is most rapid during inspiration when decreasing intrapleural pressure assists venous return to the heart. The supine posture facilitates right ventricle filling, because flow is not retarded by gravity. Right ventricular filling causes the Y descent. (**Ref. 1,** pp. 410–412)

431. (**B**) Drugs that have a positive inotropic action on the heart decrease the PEP/LVET ratio and increase ejection fraction, left ventricle maximum dP/dt, and V_{max}. (**Ref. 1,** pp. 431–434)

432. (**E**) Cardiac hypertrophy may be "physiological" (i.e., adaptive) or "pathological" (maladaptive). The increased heart mass and

enhanced functional characteristics of an athlete's heart is an example of physiological hypertrophy. (**Ref. 2,** p. 69; **Ref. 3,** p. 261)

433. **(B)** The Frank-Starling mechanism (Law of the Heart) involves a change in cardiac performance as a function of pre-load or stretch of the cardiac muscle prior to contraction. Its basis is the length-tension curve of muscle and, as such, the mechanism is intrinsic to the heart. A Frank-Starling curve defines a single inotropic state of the heart; altered contractility can only be achieved by moving to another curve, upward and to the left or downward and to the right. (**Ref. 1,** pp. 425–429)

434. **(E)** Ventricular function curves express the functional ability of the heart at a time when the data for such curves were determined. Thus, the curves represent a relationship between right atrial pressure at the input of the heart and cardiac output from the left ventricle. Each curve indicates that at any given right atrial pressure (venous return) the output increases in response to such variation in atrial filling or pressure. The degree of change depends on the conditional state of the heart. When conditions do change, as in failure (curve B), the ventricular function moves to a new output–pressure (or work–length) curve. Thus, the functional ability moved from curve A to curve B. Any successful therapeutic maneuver, as with digitalis administration, will shift the cardiac function to a new curve directed upward and to the left. Since the heart can shift from one function curve to another, the physiologic (and hence clinical) functional activity of the heart can be portrayed by a family of curves (i.e., a family of Starling law curves), with each curve corresponding to a specific set of circumstances. (**Ref. 1,** pp. 425–429)

435. **(A)** Measures of pre-load were decreased (end-diastolic volume, end-diastolic radius) whereas mean ejection pressure (a good measure of afterload) was increased markedly. Stroke volume, the difference between end-diastolic volume and end-systolic volume, was decreased. Mean arterial blood pressure was increased as evidenced by the increase in mean ejection pressure. Ventricular dilatation did not occur, as indicated by the values for end-diastolic volume and radius. (**Ref. 1,** pp. 428–429)

436. **(A)** Standing up causes blood to pool in the abdomen and legs, decreasing venous return to the heart. This decreased ventricular preload decreases diastolic stretching of the ventricle, and based

on the Frank-Starling mechanism produces decreased performance during a subsequent contraction. (**Ref. 1,** pp. 425–426)

437. **(C)** Increased inotropicity resulting from sympathetic nerve stimulation and catecholamine release moves the ventricular function curve upward and to the left. This permits increased performance at the same or smaller pre-load state. Increased ventricular pre-loading by whatever mechanism, while increasing strength of contraction, does not augment inotropic state. Decreased heart rate and heart failure result in decreased inotropic state. (**Ref. 1,** pp. 425–428)

438. **(A)** This line is shifted upward and to the left, by definition a higher inotropic state (i.e., increased contractility). (**Ref. 1,** pp. 428–429)

439. **(B)** Stimulation of cardiac adrenergic sympathetic neurons increase conduction velocity through the bundle branches and Purkinje fibers (dromotropicity), contributing to a shortening of the R-R interval. It also decreases refractoriness of the AV node, increases the rate of change of left ventricular pressure, increases stroke work, and decreases ventricular end-systolic volume. (**Ref. 1,** pp. 418–420, 434–435)

440. **(B)** Oxygen is added to blood passing through the lung, causing a negative arteriovenous oxygen (A-V_{O_2}) concentration difference. In contrast, the A-V_{O_2} concentration difference in all other organs is positive where oxygen is removed. (**Ref. 1,** pp. 547–548)

441. **(B)** Arteriovenous oxygen (A-V_{O_2}) difference across the right thigh decreased as indicated by the blood oxygen content values for right femoral artery and vein, whereas coronary vessel A-V_{O_2} difference increased (femoral artery minus coronary sinus). Ventricular pre-load increased, as judged by end-diastolic volume, as did minute work since it is a function of mean ejection pressure and heart rate (both of which increased). (**Ref. 1,** pp. 407–408)

442. **(D)** Using the Fick equation: cardiac = oxygen consumption/ (artery O_2 content − mixed ventricle O_2 content) or 150/(.20 − 0.14) or 150/.06 = 2500 ml/min. (**Ref. 1,** pp. 413–415)

443. **(C)** Oxygen utilization, or that oxygen actually used by the tissue, is a function of the blood flow rate and the arteriovenous oxygen (A-V$_{O_2}$) difference. As such, oxygen utilization must always be less than oxygen delivery. Oxygen utilization of the heart is increased by inotropic state, heart rate, afterload, and the like; however, since oxygen extraction of the heart is high and near maximal under basal conditions, little additional oxygen can be gained by further increases in A-V$_{O_2}$ difference. The only other means available is through increased flow. (**Ref. 1,** pp. 510–517)

444. **(C)** A-V$_{O_2}$ difference, the difference between arterial (A) and venous blood (E), is greatest for myocardium (B) and least for kidney (D). C is skeletal muscle. (**Ref. 1,** p. 516)

445. **(A)** Maximal heart rate is not significantly affected by endurance exercise training. (**Ref. 1,** pp. 306–307)

446. **(B)** Exercise and physical work are accompanied by a decrease in parasympathetic tone to the heart and increased sympathetic tone, increasing heart rate and inotropic state. The latter increases the rate of shortening and relaxation, increasing stroke volume and ejection fraction, decreasing ventricular end-systolic volume, and moving the Frank-Starling or ventricular function curve upward and to the left. Increased oxygen utilization in contracting skeletal muscle increases A-V$_{O_2}$ difference. (**Ref. 1,** pp. 504–505)

447. **(B)** Since blood spends most of its time traveling through the veins, circulation time is more dependent upon what happens there (e.g., venomotion) than in other vascular components.(**Ref. 2,** p. 531)

448. **(B)** A-V$_{O_2}$ difference was increased across the coronary vessels. The medication decreased, not increased, the A-V$_{O_2}$ difference across the right thigh. Left ventricular pre-load was increased as judged from end-diastolic volume, and afterload was increased based on mean ejection pressure. (**Ref. 1,** pp. 407–408)

449. **(D)** C is oxygen consumption while at rest. D is reserve oxygen consumption at a high work rate. F is residual oxygen delivery, not usable by the tissues. A minus B is A-V$_{O_2}$ difference under resting conditions. (**Ref. 1,** pp. 410–411)

450. (A) Coronary vascular resistance in the left ventricle increases during the time the ventricle is contracting due to the squeezing action of the muscle on the blood in the lumina and on the tissue itself, thus limiting blood flow during that period of the cardiac cycle. Coronary flow may increase four to sixfold with increased work demand, as determined by heart rate, inotropic state, wall stress, and several minor factors. Because flow is dependent primarily upon the difference between arterial blood pressure and ventricular luminal (i.e., tissue) pressure, incomplete relaxation impedes overall coronary flow. **(Ref. 1,** pp. 510–517)

451. (D) Stimulation of beta-1 adrenergic receptors in the heart increases inotropic state, heart rate, and conduction velocity. The first two act powerfully to increase myocardial oxygen demand, which through local control mechanisms, decrease coronary vascular resistance and coronary flow. Decreased coronary perfusion pressure may or may not decrease coronary flow depending upon position in the autoregulatory range. Increased ventricular diastolic pressure increase coronary vascular resistance, thus decreasing coronary flow. Beta-2 adrenergic receptor stimulation in the heart has little influence on coronary flow. **(Ref. 1,** pp. 510–517)

452. (D) Ischemia is a condition of oxygen deprivation accompanied by the inadequate supply/removal of other metabolites consequent to reduced blood flow. Indications are an abnormally increased A-VO_2 difference at rest, elevated coronary A-V lactate, and release of various marker enzymes (LDH, CPK). Electrocardiographically, coronary ischemia is characterized by acute changes in the ST segment and T wave. **(Ref. 1,** pp. 515–516)

453. (B) Vasodilation is maximal at point B. Further fall in perfusion pressure is accompanied by decrease in flow. The autoregulatory range extends from B to D. Vasoconstriction is maximal at D and flow increases sharply beyond it if perfusion pressure increases further. **(Ref. 1,** pp. 511–512)

454. (C) Blood returning from the placenta through the umbilical veins, having just received oxygen from maternal blood, has the highest oxygen content and percent saturation. **(Ref. 1,** pp. 527–529)

455. (A)   Left-shift of the ODC of human fetal blood is much smaller than that of the lamb relative to their respective mothers' blood. Fetal acidosis usually right-shifts the ODC (Bohr effect), resulting in a smaller difference in affinities between the two bloods. Increasing maternal alkalosis acts to decrease the difference between the positions of the ODCs of the fetus and the mother. The normal human p50 is about 26 mm Hg. (**Ref. 1,** pp. 527–529)

456. (C)   Hypoxia produces an effect in the fetus similar to the adult diving response (i.e., bradycardia). (**Ref. 1,** pp. 527–529)

457. (C)   Venous blood of low oxygen saturation is seen in the inferior vena cava and the right atrium. Venous blood should also be seen in the right ventricle and the pulmonary artery. The unexpected increase from 68% saturation to 83% between the right atrium and the right ventricle is known as an "oxygen step-up." It indicates the leakage of arterial blood into the right ventricle. The most likely condition which would cause this is a ventricular septal defect, a left to right shunt. (**Ref. 1,** pp. 527–529)

458. (C)   Functional foramen ovale closure is primarily a function of increased pulmonary flow and venous return to the left atrium. Shunting through the ductus arteriosus reverses shortly after birth, coursing from the aorta to the pulmonary artery as aortic pressure rises above that of the pulmonary artery. The sudden fall in pulmonary vascular resistance is a function of rising lung pO_2, experienced after the first breath. (**Ref. 1,** pp. 527–529)

459. (D)   In a fashion analogous to Ohm's Law ($R = E/I$), vascular resistance is a function of perfusion pressure and flow rate. It is often expressed in peripheral resistance units (PRU). Without knowing flow, resistance cannot be determined from the pressure change alone. As in an electrical circuit, the total resistance of several resistances in series is equal to their sum. The venous side of the systemic circulation usually represents less than 10% of total peripheral resistance. The pulmonary circulation has less than one-fifth the resistance of the systemic circulation. (**Ref. 1,** pp. 443–446)

460. (C)   Two requirements for rigorous adherence to the Poiseuille equation is laminar (streamline) flow and Newtonian flow characteristics (i.e., viscosity independent of flow velocity and shear rate and of tube caliber). (**Ref. 1,** pp. 441–443)

461. (E) In this diagram the flow is streamline in nature with the fluid in lamina A having the greatest velocity. The velocity of flow in lamina B is greater than in C, which is faster than in D. In fact, the fluid layer in D, which is in contact with the vessel wall, moves barely or does not move at all. Most of the red blood cells flow in the fastest layers, which will be in the center. The highest the pressure is exerted against the wall, at the wall, not out in the stream of flow. **(Ref. 1,** pp. 446–448)

462. (B) Perfusion pressure is the difference between transmural pressures at two different sites in an hydraulic system, and along with velocity (kinetic energy) is responsible for moving fluid from the one site to another. Because venous pressure at the heart is normally only a few mm Hg, perfusion pressure of the systemic circulation is usually equal to, or slightly less, than the mean arterial pressure. Perfusion pressure of the coronary circulation is greatly influenced by ventricular luminal pressure. Perfusion pressure is not influenced by gravity because its effects on transmural pressure are equivalent in arteries and veins at the same level in the body. **(Ref. 1,** pp. 438–440)

463. (C) Vasodilation decreases vascular resistance, while increased cardiac output causes an increase in blood pressure. Vasoconstriction is incompatible with a decrease in vascular resistane, with or without change in cardiac output. Vasodilation and decrease in cardiac output would further exacerbate any fall in blood pressure. Decrease in venous return to the heart would result from vasoconstriction, and would decrease cardiac output. **(Ref. 1,** pp. 443–446)

464. (D) In the Fahraeus effect, the dynamic hematocrit falls well below the bulk hematocrit in small vessels, both because of erythrocyte screening and the higher velocity of the erythrocytes traveling near the tube axis. The plasma moves more slowly near the wall. The Fahraeus effect is the major explanation for the Fahraeus-Lindqvist effect, whereby viscosity decreases in blood flowing through small vessels. Neither phenomena occur with Newtonian fluids (e.g., water). **(Ref. 1,** pp. 448–451)

465. (C) When blood begins to move under the influence of pressure, the erythrocytes move away from the wall toward the tube axis. They become oriented with respect to each other and the wall and move at a higher velocity than the cell-free plasma along the wall.

In so doing, the viscosity of the fluid near the wall is decreased, as is the dynamic viscosity of the whole blood column. Blood flowing through small tubes shows a lower hematocrit and thus viscosity than when flowing in larger tubes, a phenomenon known as the Sigma or Fahraeus-Lindqvist effect. This results from both the relatively larger cell-free volume in the smaller tubes and the exclusion of some fraction of erythrocytes from small tubes. The Sigma effect does not apply to capillaries; viscosity increases sharply in tubes of less than 5 to 7 μm because of the erythrocyte deformation required for passage. (**Ref. 1**, pp. 448–451)

466. (B) In systems in which gravity can be disregarded, total fluid energy is equal to the potential energy (pressure) plus the kinetic energy (velocity). Although the pressure component is predominant in most situations in the circulation, kinetic energy comes to assume a significant fraction of fluid energy in the veins, especially in the largest veins. Fluid energy is highest in the large arteries and lowest in the large veins, thus the impetus for fluid movement through the circulatory tree. Fluid energy is dissipated against friction in the cardiovascular system, not against gravity. This is because the circulation is a closed circuit, blood going up comes down, and vice versa like a siphon. The Poiseuille equation involves expressions of perfusion pressure, viscosity, radius, and so on, but no expression of fluid energy. (**Ref. 1**, pp. 438–441)

467. (E) The Poiseuille equation states that flow is directly proportional to perfusion pressure, inversely proportional to fluid viscosity; directly proportional to radius raised to the fourth power, and inversely proportional to vessel length. Thus, as perfusion pressure increases, flow increases directly. On the other hand, as viscosity rises, flow decreases directly. The most powerful factor determining fluid flow and the one most significant to blood flow in tissue is radius. This is the case because blood vessels are capable of changing their caliber by contraction and relaxation of smooth muscle: radius is raised to the fourth power. Thus a tiny change in radius results in a large change in flow. The Poiseuille equation only applies for streamline flow and for non-distensible tubes. (**Ref. 1**, pp. 441–443)

468. (C) As a result of the elastic properties of the blood vascular wall, the size of the vessel lumen is a function of the forces applied to it. In the normal system, alteration in the dimension of most blood vessels along their longitudinal axis is only slight. However, changes in vessel circumference commonly occur *in vivo* and this important relationship between pressure, wall tension, and the diameter of the elastic tube was expressed by LaPlace as $T = Pr$. The pressure, P, which is physiologically relevant, is the force acting radially on each unit area of the wall and includes the intraluminal pressure (P_I), as well as the pressure which is affecting the external surface of the vessel (P_E). This transmural pressure (P_T), which is exerted on the vessel wall, is the difference between internal and external pressure ($P_T = P_I - P_E$). This relationship usually operates in blood vessels with very thin walls and when wall thickness is increased, as with age or disease; then the pressure–tension relationship becomes extremely complex and clinically relevant. (**Ref. 1,** pp. 466–467)

469. (A) The veins, including the venules, small veins, large veins and venous sinuses, and the vena cavae normally contain 60% to 70% of the total blood volume. (**Ref. 1,** pp. 361–363)

470. (C) At rest, the arterioles normally account for about 40% of total vascular resistance, and the capillaries approximately 25%. The aorta, vena cavae, and terminal veins each account for less than 5% of total resistance. (**Ref. 1,** pp. 361–363)

471. (A) The Windkessel effect most greatly dampens pulse pressure in the aorta and large arteries, whose elastic walls store pressure (potential) energy during ventricular systole. There is little if any pulse pressure in capillaries and venules, so no Windkessel effect. (**Ref. 1,** pp. 361–363)

472. (C) Total resistance is calculated in the same way as in an electrical circuit. (**Ref. 1,** pp. 443–445)

473. (C) Bed rest, space flight, and alcohol consumption all cause vascular smooth muscle to relax, increasing venous wall compliance. (**Ref. 1,** pp. 454–456)

474. (C) Due to arterial wall aging and atherosclerotic processes arterial wall compliance decreases, producing less hydraulic dampening, hence an increased pulse pressure. (**Ref. 1,** p. 456)

475. (B) Wall tension is equal to transmural pressure times radius. **(Ref. 1,** pp. 466–467)

476. (B) Critical closure pressure is the perfusion pressure at which flow through a vascular bed ceases. It is dependent upon the tone of vascular smooth muscle, which, in turn, is dependent on neural and hormonal input to the vascular bed as well as intrinsic blood flow control mechanisms. **(Ref. 1,** pp. 481–483, 511–512)

477. (C) Skeletal muscle arterioles contain both alpha- and beta-adrenergic receptors, the former producing constriction and the latter, dilation. Cutaneous vasodilation is primarily a function of decreased alpha-adrenergic receptor stimulation. Heart rate is mainly a function of increased beta-1 adrenergic receptor stimulation. **(Ref. 1,** pp. 513–514)

478. (B) Angiotensin II inhibits renin release. **(Ref. 1,** pp. 772–775)

479. (A) The direct hemodynamic effect of an increase in heart rate is to decrease pulse pressure since less time is available for "run-off." Thus, decreased heart rate increases pulse pressure. Factors increasing pulse pressure are increased stroke volume and decreased arterial compliance and vascular resistance. **(Ref. 1,** pp. 460–462)

480. (A) The direct effect of norepinephrine on the heart is to increase rate, inortopicity and dromotropicity. Increased arterial blood pressure resulting from peripheral vasoconstriction due to the effect of norepinephrine on alpha-receptors, reflexly suppresses heart rate. Depression of the CNS, as resulting from anesthetic treatment, prevents this reflex suppression. **(Ref. 1,** pp. 537–540)

481. (B) The carotid sinus baroreceptors are receptors sensitive to stretch (indirectly pressure) which are located in the walls of the common carotid artery at its bifurcation. As vessel pressure increases above 40 mm Hg, receptor firing rate increases. They are more sensitive to rising pressure than to constant pressure. Maximal firing rate is reached at about 180 mm Hg. The carotid sinus receptors are more sensitive and have a greater effect on rapid blood pressure control than the aortic receptors or other receptors. The reflex effect of falling pressure is to decrease firing rate, which reflexly decreases parasympathetic tone to the heart, increasing the heart rate. **(Ref. 1,** pp. 538–540)

482. (B) Central blood volume (volume in the heart, lungs, and associated great vessels) strongly influences blood volume control, stroke volume, and arterial blood pressure. Central blood volume is increased by blood volume expansion (e.g., transfusion), microgravity or weightlessness, negative G force, lower body immersion in water, and lower body positive pressure. Central blood volume is decreased by standing upright from a lying down position (orthostasis), positive pressure breathing, positive G force, lower body negative pressure, and the Valsalva maneuver. **(Ref. 1,** pp. 506–507)

483. (B) Blood volume increases sharply during pregnancy mainly as the result of an increase in plasma volume. Uterine blood flow increases manyfold. Cardiac output increases as the result of increases in both heart rate and stroke volume. Pregnant women hyperventilate, particularly during late gestation. This leads to some degree of alkalosis, increasing the production of 2,3-diphosphoglycerate (2,3-DPG) by the erythrocyte. **(Ref. 1,** pp. 527–529)

484. (D) Increased osmolality of the extracellular compartment associated with a reduction in volume will inhibit the cardiac volume receptors and stimulate the hypothalamic osmoreceptors resulting in an increase in ADH secretion, thus conserving water. **(Ref. 1,** pp. 759–762)

485. (A) Fluid movement = k $[(P_c + \pi i) - (P_i + \pi p)]$ or $[(25 + 10) - (3 + 30)]$ or $[35 - 33] = +2$. Thus the net tendency is for filtration. **(Ref. 1,** pp. 472–475)

486. (B) Riva Rocci developed the indirect method of measuring arterial blood pressure using the sphygmomanometer. Karl Ludwig invented the recording instrument known as the kymograph. Corneille Heymans is credited with first demonstrating the vasomotor reflexes. **(Ref. 1,** pp. 412–413)

487. (C) When blood pressure rises, the heart rate falls and vice versa. **(Ref. 1,** pp. 538–539)

488. (B) Heart rate is reflexly depressed in stage 1 because of transiently elevated arterial blood pressure. Increased mouth/intrapleural pressure assists left ventricle ejection, momentarily increasing blood pressure. **(Ref. 1,** pp. 507–508)

489. **(C)** External water (hydrostatic) pressure has no influence on the extent to which the diving reflex is expressed. (**Ref. 1,** pp. 599–611)

490. **(D)** Endurance exercise augments the capacity of the veins to increase tone during orthostatic maneuvers. All the other conditions decrease this capacity. Denervation of the carotid and aortic baroreceptors destroys the capability of the baroreflex to respond to orthostatic changes. (**Ref. 1,** pp. 506–507)

491. **(D)** Dizziness ensues during hyperventilation because CO_2 is blown off, causing cerebral vasoconstriction, decreased blood perfusion, and cerebral hypoxemia since too little oxygen reaches the brain. (**Ref. 1,** p. 559)

492. **(B)** During inspiration, intrapleural pressure decreases, increasing right heart venous return and pre-load. This increases right ventricle stroke volume through the Frank-Starling mechanism. Blood reaching the lungs, however, tends to stay in the lungs as the air and blood capacity is increasing. This decreases venous return, hence pre-load in the left ventricle. Increased right ventricle pre-load also moves the interventricular septum to the left, limiting left ventricle filling capacity. The net result is a decrease in left ventricle stroke volume and, therefore, a momentary fall in arterial blood pressure. A rapid reflex increase in heart rate via the medullary cardiovascular centers ensues as parasympathetic inhibition of the heart is relieved and sympathetic drive is increased. Reflex arterial/arteriolar constriction would also be expected to occur in order to maintain blood pressure constant as blood pressure falls, but this effect is modest. Also, an increased firing of pulmonary stretch (Hering-Breuer) receptors takes place with inspiration, which send their information to the medullary respiratory center. These, in turn, "cross-talk" to the nearby medullary cardiovascular centers amplifying the cardiac speeding. (**Ref. 1,** pp. 604–606)

493. **(B)** Bleeding time is the time necessary for a small nick to stop bleeding (2 to 3 min). This measurement is normal in hemophilia because the cessation of bleeding is due to the plugging of the wound by platelets which is normal in hemophilia. In hemophilia the coagulation time (but not bleeding time) is usually prolonged because the thromboplastin activity is abnormal. (**Ref. 1,** pp. 339–340)

494. (D) The primary pacemaker of the heart is the SA node. Activity originating from any other site represents an abnormal situation, usually such "secondary" pacemaker activity resides within the Purkinje system. (**Ref. 1,** pp. 376–381)

495. (B) Tetany can occur in skeletal muscle because several contractile events can be summated. The long electrical refractory period of cardiac muscle precludes this possibility. (**Ref. 1,** pp. 368–375)

496. (B) Aortic flow velocity reaches a maximum during the early rapid phase of ventricular ejection and then decreases. (**Ref. 1,** pp. 407–408)

497. (C) If large regions of abnormally low V/Q ratio do exist, there will be a shunt of blood past the oxygenation mechanism of the lungs. This will result in both cyanosis and systemic arterial blood hypoxemia. (**Ref. 1,** pp. 584–589)

498. (E) The blood pressure found in the main pulmonary artery is not inversely proportional to lung tissue or the cardiac output. Also, alveolar hypoxia does not result in vasodilation; indeed, vasoconstriction may occur. Pulmonary artery pressure is not always high enough to perfuse the top of the human lungs. (**Ref. 2,** pp. 534–536)

499. (A) The area of the pressure–volume diagram is a very close approximation of cardiac work. (**Ref. 2,** pp. 514–517)

500. (B) Coronary vasodilation is the normal response to cardiac sympathetic stimulation. (**Ref. 2,** pp. 547–550)

501. (C) The myogenic theory of autoregulation of blood flow proposes that flow to a tissue bed is kept constant when pressure increases because of an inherent adjustment of smooth muscle to stretch. (**Ref. 2,** pp. 566–567)

502. (D) Venoconstriction adds to a redistribution of blood and increased cardiac output during exercise. (**Ref. 2,** pp. 577–579)

503. (B) Flow through a rigid tube is related inversely to the first power of the length of that tube. (**Ref. 2,** pp. 530–532)

504. (B) In normal ranges, as the diastolic volume of the heart increases the force and the rate of contraction of cardiac muscle fibers will increase. (**Ref. 2,** pp. 520–521)

505. (B) A rigid aorta will accommodate less blood during ejection, thereby raising the resistance to movement of blood out of the heart. (**Ref. 2,** pp. 532–544)

506. (B) A patient with the signs listed has normal function except for the increased blood pressure. This indicates hypertension. (**Ref. 2,** pp. 585–588)

507. (A) Any condition that increases blood pooling contributes to congestive heart failure. This would include decreased arterial pressure, increased serum sodium, and increased tissue hydrostatic pressure. (**Ref. 2,** pp. 588–589)

508. (C) During exercise, the greatest portion of additional oxygen supplied to working tissues comes from an increase in arteriovenous oxygen difference. (**Ref. 2,** pp. 577–579)

509. (A) The aorta displays the greatest Windkessel effect. (**Ref. 2,** p. 533)

510. (C) A blood oxygen saturation of 73% in a normal individual would indicate a sampling site in a vein. Systolic and diastolic pressures of 28 mm Hg and 15 mm Hg, respectively, are found only in the pulmonary artery. *Note:* Right ventricle diastolic pressure is close to zero. (**Ref. 2,** pp. 515–517)

511. (F) Usually vasovagal syncope occurs in two phases. First, blood pressure falls as the result of hypovolemia, orthostasis, venous pooling, and the like with little reflex change in cardiac output or forearm venous tone, although the heart rate may increase. Following this, the "C" afferent fibers from the cardiopulmonary receptors become active, resulting in intensified parasympathetic tone to the heart, causing bradycardia, and decreasing sympathetic tone to the periphery, producing vasodilatation and a fall in arterial blood pressure. The resulting cerebral hypoperfusion causes a greying-out or a blacking-out and the associated diaphoresis and nausea. (**Ref. 2,** pp. 584–585)

512. **(G)** In phase II of the Valsalva maneuver, venous return to the heart is decreased as the result of elevated intrapleural pressure, reducing ventricular pre-load, hence stroke volume and blood pressure. The latter is responsible for reflexly raising heart rate. This phase may continue for many seconds with both the hypotension and the tachycardia becoming progressively more extreme. **(Ref. 2,** pp. 551–552)

513. **(B)** $CO = mL/min$ of O_2 used/AV-O_2 mL/min = 5.51 L/min. **(Ref. 2,** pp. 518–519)

514. **(A)** Stroke volume = CO mL/min / heart beats/min = 55 mL/beat. **(Ref. 2,** pp. 518–519)

515. **(E)** CO = heart rate × stroke volume = 10.5 L/min **(Ref. 2,** pp. 518–519)

516. **(A)** **(Ref. 2,** pp. 520–521)

517. **(B)** **(Ref. 2,** pp. 520–521)

518. **(C)** **(Ref. 2,** pp. 533–534)

519. **(D)** **(Ref. 2,** pp. 533–534, 536–540)

520. **(D)** The mean blood pressure decreases as the blood moves from the aorta into capillaries. Because of the inverse relationship between flow velocity and cross-sectional area, the blood flows much more slowly in the distal arteries and especially in the arterioles with the lowest velocity in the capillaries. This permits the greatest fluid, nutrients, and waste product exchange. The resistance to flow is determined largely by the blood viscosity and radius. (Hence, the viscosity in the capillaries is less than in the arterioles.) The greatest resistance to flow is in the arterioles. **(Ref. 2,** pp. 533–534)

521. **(C)** Approximately .16 seconds after the onset of the P wave, the QRS waves appear as a result of depolarization of the ventricles. **(Ref. 2,** p. 516)

522. **(E)** The atrial C wave occurs because of the bulging of the AV valves toward the atria. This comes about because of the increascing pressure in the ventricles and pulling on the atrial muscle where it is attached to the ventricular muscle by the contracting ventricles. (**Ref. 2**, p. 516)

523. **(F)** As soon as systole is over and the ventricular pressures fall again to their low diastolic values, the high pressures in the atria immediately push the AV valves open and allow blood to flow rapidly into the ventricles. (**Ref. 2**, p. 516)

524. **(D)** The T wave represents the stage of repolarization of the ventricles at the time the ventricular muscles begin to relax. (**Ref. 2**, p. 516)

525. **(B)** At the end of systole, ventricular relaxation begins suddenly allowing the intraventricular pressures in the large arteries to immediately push blood back toward the ventricles, which snaps the aortic and pulmonary valves closed. (**Ref. 2**, p. 516)

526. **(A)** When ventricular contraction is over the AV valves open, allowing blood to flow rapidly into the ventricles. (**Ref. 2**, p. 516)

527. **(A)** The first heart sound is largely due to closure of the atrioventricular valves and coincides with the period of isovolumetric contraction. (**Ref. 2**, pp. 517–518)

528. **(D)** The Q wave of the ECG immediately precedes isovolumic contraction. (**Ref. 2**, pp. 516–517)

529. **(E)** The T wave of the ECG occurs during the period of ventricular ejection. (**Ref. 2**, pp. 516–517)

530. **(C)** The P wave of the ECG is due to depolarization of the atria and immediately precedes atrial contraction. (**Ref. 2**, pp. 516–517)

531. **(B)** During the period of isovolumetric relaxation the second heart sound can be heard. (**Ref. 2**, pp. 516–517)

532. **(B)** Mean arterial pressure is decreased by aortic regurgitation and mitral stenosis. Aortic regurgitation is caused by the return of blood from the elastic aorta through the defective valve during diastole. Mitral stenosis is an obstruction to the flow through the

orifice so that blood must be forced from the atrium during diastole. Both result in arterial pressure. (**Ref. 2,** p. 518)

533. (**A**)   In aortic regurgitation, return of blood from the aorta
through the defective valve causes increased left atrial pressure.
(In mitral valve stenosis, there is an obstruction to blood flow
from the atrium also resulting in increased atrial pressure.) (**Ref.
2,** p. 518)

534. (**B**)   In aortic regurgitation, return of the blood through the defective valve causes a decreased volume of blood pumped into systemic
circulation, thus a decreased cardiac output is caused. In mitral stenosis, there is a decreased volume of blood pumped into the left ventricle resulting in decreased cardiac output. (**Ref. 2,** p. 518)

535. (**A**)   In aortic regurgitation, there is increased blood return to the
left ventricle by the defective valve with resulting increased left
ventricular volume. In mitral stenosis, there is decreased filling of
the left ventricle resulting in increased left atrial blood volume.
(**Ref. 2,** p. 518)

536. (**A**)   In aortic regurgitation, there is increased return of blood
through the defective valve to increase left ventricular volume. In
mitral stenosis, there is a decreased filling of the left ventricle by
the defective valve, resulting in decreased left ventricular volume.
(**Ref. 2,** p. 518)

537. (**A**)   In aortic regurgitation, there is decreased cardiac output, as
is true in mitral stenosis due to defective valves. This results in
decreased peripheral flow which envokes a compensatory reflex.
Renal output slows down until blood volume increases. (**Ref. 2,**
p. 518)

538. (**A**)   It is the first electrical event recorded on the ECG and represents atrial depolarization. (**Ref. 2,** pp. 500–504)

539. (**H**)   Represents part of the ventricular depolarization the wave-
front goes down the septum. (**Ref. 2,** pp. 500–504)

540. (J)   Represents the major vector of ventricular depolarization. (Ref. 2, pp. 500–504)

541. (I)   The terminal portion of ventricular depolarization. (Ref. 2, pp. 500–504)

542. (C)   A ventricular muscle repolarization (phase 3 of the action potential). (Ref. 2, pp. 500–504)

543. (B)   May be the representation of Purkinje fiber repolarization and/or afterpotentials. (Ref. 2, pp. 500–504)

544. (E)   The time during which the impulse activates the atria and passes through the AV node and specialized conducting system. (Ref. 2, pp. 500–504)

545. (D)   The complete or total representation of ventricular muscle depolarization. (Ref. 2, p. 500–504)

546. (F)   Terminal ventricular depolarization to onset of repolarization is temporally equal to the phase 2 of ventricular muscle action potentials. (Ref. 2, pp. 500–504)

547. (G)   The entire period of time of ventricular repolarization includes phases 2 and 3 of ventricular muscle action potentials. (Ref. 2, pp. 500–504)

Summary of answers 538–547: The ECG deflections comprise four positive and three negative waves. Some of these waves are termed "complexes" when they are combined and all are descriptive, indicating some specific physiologic event(s) occurring in the heart. The waves, the various intervals and segments, provide a way of measuring the direction of a specific event. Both the contours and polarity of the complexes recorded from each lead of the ECG depend on the orientation of the excitation fronts of the heart. (Ref. 2, pp. 500–504)

7

Endocrine Physiology

MULTIPLE CHOICE

DIRECTIONS (Questions 548–617): Each of the questions or incomplete statements below is followed by five suggested answers or completions. Select the **one** that is **best** in each case.

548. Insulin
- **A.** decreases fatty acid synthesis
- **B.** is necessary for the storage of foodstuffs during a meal
- **C.** has no effect on fatty acid metabolism
- **D.** is necessary for glycogenolysis
- **E.** B and D are correct

549. After the first 5 months of pregnancy
- **A.** uterine engorgement is maintained by placental estrogen and progesterone
- **B.** low levels of estrogen inhibit further ovulation
- **C.** FSH maintains a normal rate of follicular maturation
- **D.** uterine engorgement is maintained by follicular estrogen and progesterone
- **E.** A and C are correct

550. The action of parathormone on the kidney tends to
  A. effectively increase the deposition of bone mineral
  B. increase calcium phosphate precipitation in the kidney
  C. elevate serum phosphate
  D. diminish the possibility of hyperphosphatemia
  E. A and C are correct

551. Glucocorticoid hormones from the adrenal cortex
  A. increase the concentrations of enzymes necessary for glucose synthesis
  B. mobilize fatty acids from muscle
  C. decrease glucose formation in the liver
  D. increase the movement of amino acids from the blood into most cells of the body
  E. all are correct

552. Parathyroid hormone
  A. decreases urinary excretion of Ca^{2+}
  B. increases Ca^{2+} release from bone
  C. A and B are correct
  D. decreases Ca^{2+} release from bone
  E. all are correct

553. Serum cholesterol is elevated by
  A. ingestion of dietary fatty acids
  B. ingestion of dietary cholesterol
  C. obstruction of the common bile duct
  D. reabsorption and recirculation of bile acids
  E. all are correct

554. Abnormally low concentrations of estrogen result in
  A. lack of or very late appearance of pubic hair
  B. increased deposition of fat in the subcutaneous area
  C. increased retention of Na^+ and water
  D. decreased height
  E. all are correct

555. The function of the endocrine system includes which of the following?
   A. Body weight and size
   B. Regulation of growth and maturation
   C. Behavior of the organism and its reproduction
   D. Regulation of metabolic substrates and mineral flow for maintenance of chemical homeostasis
   E. All are correct

556. Which of the following is considered true regarding the endocrine system versus the neural system?
   A. Both transmit signals that are widespread and diverse
   B. Both transmit signals that are highly focused and localized
   C. A and B are correct
   D. The two systems differ only in their modes for transmission of chemical signals
   E. All are correct

557. The neurocrine mechanism may be characterized by
   A. a mechanism of transmission that includes the circulatory system
   B. a concept of a "neurohormone"
   C. A and B are correct
   D. the relatively short distance involved during the transmission of messenger molecules
   E. all are correct

558. According to the neuroendocrine system concept, a messenger molecule may function as a(an)
   A. paracrine and autocrine hormone
   B. endocrine and neurotransmitter
   C. A and B are correct
   D. endocrine hormone only
   E. all are correct

559. Which of the following is considered true regarding hormone synthesis?

A. Co-peptide synthesis and secretion parallel hormone synthesis and release

B. Mature messenger RNA directs the synthesis of a preprohormone peptide sequence on ribosomes, after which the N-terminal signal is removed and the resultant peptide is transferred vectorially into the endoplasmic reticulum

C. Final cleavage of the prohormone takes place in the secretory granules and the Golgi apparatus, where it is then stored in granules ready for secretion by exocytosis

D. Nuclear posttranscriptional modification of the primary gene transcript includes excision of introns, splicing of exons, capping of the 5' end, and addition of poly-A at the 3' end

E. All are correct

560. Catecholamine and protein hormones are characterized as having the following properties

A. mobilized as a result of stimuli that usually raise cytosolic potassium ion levels along with increased levels of intracellular ATP

B. mobilized as a result of stimuli that lower intracellular cAMP with a concomitant rise in cytosolic calcium ions

C. utilize secretory granules for storage and transport to cell membrane for exocytosis into the extracellular space

D. simple compartmentalization with subsequent transfer of the free cytosolic form through the plasma membrane

E. A and C are correct

561. One mode of hormone synthesis and release involves the modification of hormone X from cell X by adjacent cell Y to produce hormone Y. This mode is typical of

A. adrenalin hormone synthesis

B. estrogen hormone synthesis

C. vitamin D hormone synthesis

D. angiotensin hormone synthesis

E. none are correct

562. Chronotropic control is a general mechanism for governing hormone secretion. Typical examples of chronotropic control are
   A. menstrual rhythm
   B. sleep–wake cycle
   C. seasonal rhythm
   D. developmental rhythm
   E. all are correct

563. Assuming that "product" is a function of hormone secretion, which of the following is(are) associated with the principle of negative feedback control of hormone secretion?
   A. Hormone secretion may be inhibited by a deficit in product serum levels
   B. Hormone secretion may be stimulated by a deficit in product serum levels
   C. Increased product from target cell suppresses further hormone secretion
   D. Increase in hormone secretion stimulates a greater output of product from a target cell
   E. All are correct

564. Receptors for steroid hormones
   A. are located in the cytosol
   B. are located in the nucleus
   C. A and B are correct
   D. are relatively small protein molecules ranging in number from 20 to 100 per cell
   E. all are correct

565. With increasing concentration of hormone in solution with a fixed number of cells, the amount of bound hormone
   A. increases until bound hormone equals the K value for the association, assuming free hormone concentration approaches infinity
   B. to free hormone ratio approaches 0, assuming free hormone concentration approaches infinity
   C. to free hormone ratio approaches 1, assuming free hormone concentration approaches infinity
   D. increases until 50% of receptor sites are occupied
   E. B and D are correct

566. In a cell where receptor binding is rate limiting
   A. decrease in receptor affinity increases the cell's sensitivity
   B. decrease in receptor site number enhances the cell's sensitivity
   C. the maximal responsiveness of the cell to hormones is increased with an increase in receptor site number
   D. sustained levels of excess hormone concentration result in increased number of receptor sites
   E. A and C are correct

567. Which of the following is **NOT** a system for coupling hormone recognition to hormone action?
   A. Calcium-calmodulin system
   B. Membrane phospholipid system
   C. Adenylate cyclase-cAMP system
   D. Lysozymal degradation system
   E. None of the above

568. Which is **NOT** a feature of the adenylate cyclase-cAMP system?
   A. Conversion of GTP to GMP concomitant conversion of ATP to cAMP
   B. Activation of regulatory unit by GDP activates catalytic unit
   C. A and B are correct
   D. Conversion of GTP to GDP with concomitant conversion of Mg-ATP to cAMP
   E. All are correct

569. Which of the following may be said regarding the calcium-calmodulin system for the transduction of hormonal signals?
   A. Requires magnesium-specific binding protein
   B. Serves only to regulate intracellular calcium ion concentrations
   C. Serves to deactivate as well as activate various enzyme and metabolic pathways
   D. Requires specific nuclear proteins essential to creating calcium channels upon binding of hormone to receptor sites
   E. A and C are correct

570. Steroid hormones
   A. are specific for cytoplasmic receptors
   B. are specific for membrane-bound receptors
   C. produce effects fast due to their mode of transcriptional and translational regulation

D. produce effects fairly rapidly, which is typical of plasma membrane response mechanisms

E. A, B, and C are correct

571. Which of the following is **NOT** a feature of the phospholipid (phosphotidyl) system of hormone action?

A. Formation of phosphotidyl inositol-4,5-bis-phosphate

B. Release of arachidonic acid by hydrolysis of diacylglycerols serves as substrate for the synthesis of calmodulin

C. Deactivation of a non-calcium-dependent protein kinase by the action of diacylglycerol

D. Cleavage of phosphotidyl inositol-4,5-bis-phosphate by membrane-bound phospholipase

E. B and D are correct

572. Which of the following is a feature of (measurable) hormone responsivity?

A. Receptor number

B. Hormone concentration

C. Minimal threshold concentration of hormone

D. Concentration of rate-limiting enzymes, co-factors, or substrates

E. All are correct

573. Which of the following is(are) true regarding the dose-response for the action of hormones?

A. Target cells require no threshold concentration for measurable response

B. Concentration of hormone required to elicit a half-measurable response defines the sensitivity of the cell

C. A and B are correct

D. Response is generally an all-or-none phenomenon

E. All are correct

574. The extent of protein binding

A. is greater for protein hormones than thyroid/steroid hormones

B. does not affect excretion rates and half-life

C. is high for all thyroid and steroid hormones (<10%)

D. renders hormone exit into interstitial fluid irreversible

E. A and C are correct

575. Metabolic clearance rate (MCR)
   A. means clearance rate
   B. is defined as the volume of plasma cleared per unit time
   C. is the sum of all removal processes, such as urinary excretion, metabolic degradation, and target cell uptake
   D. is a measure of the efficiency with which erythrocytes are removed from the plasma
   E. none of the above

576. Under ordinary basal metabolic conditions
   A. the RQ for fat is lower than for protein
   B. the respiratory quotient (RQ) for glucose is higher than for fat
   C. fat is a minor energy source
   D. fat provides over half the daily caloric requirements
   E. B and D are correct

577. In the post-absorptive state (overnight fast) for a normal adult
   A. plasma glucose levels are 60 to 115 mg/dL
   B. the brain accounts for about 10% of all glucose utilized
   C. the significant source of glucose in post-absorptive state is hepatic gluconeogenesis
   D. glycogen is the predominant precursor for gluconeogenesis in maintaining blood glucose level
   E. A and C are correct

578. Which of the following is(are) true regarding progesterone?
   A. Produced by the ovaries
   B. Secreted by the placenta
   C. Secreted by the corpus luteum
   D. Enhances fertility
   E. A, B, and C are correct

579. Estrogens are produced by the
   A. Leydig cells of the testes
   B. ovary
   C. A and B are correct
   D. liver
   E. all are correct

580. Spermatogenesis requires
   A. follicle-stimulating hormone (FSH)
   B. androgens
   C. A and B are correct
   D. adrenocorticotropic hormone (ACTH)
   E. all are correct

581. After fertilization of the ovum the
   A. corpus luteum finally fails after about 2 weeks
   B. conceptus begins to divide in the fallopian tube
   C. corpus luteum is supported by human chorionic gonadotropin (HCG)
   D. uterine engorgement is maintained by luteal progesterone for several days
   E. all are correct

582. Secretion of glucocorticosteroids is
   A. increased by stress
   B. decreased if exogenous glucocorticosteroids are given
   C. A and B are correct
   D. decreased by ACTH
   E. all are correct

583. The physiologic action(s) of estrogen on the vagina include
   A. mucosal thickening
   B. epithelial cornification
   C. deposition of glycogen
   D. increased mitosis; growth and differentiation of mucosal layers
   E. all are correct

584. Diabetes mellitus is characterized by
   A. polyuria
   B. polydipsia
   C. glycosuria
   D. polyphagia
   E. all are correct

585. Pituitary secretion
- **A.** shows a negative feedback relationship with its target organs
- **B.** if increased will usually cause target gland atrophy
- **C.** will increase as long as target gland secretion is high
- **D.** will decrease if levels of circulating target gland secretions are low
- **E.** A and C are correct

586. The thyroid hormones
- **A.** act on discrete target organs
- **B.** do not act immediately on their target cell following their release
- **C.** act on discrete organ systems
- **D.** are necessary for maintenance of life
- **E.** B and D are correct

587. Anterior pituitary secretion
- **A.** is independent of CNS control from above the level of the hypothalamus
- **B.** of only one pituitary hormone is signaled by each hypothalamic-releasing factor
- **C.** depends on a direct neural connection between the hypothalamus and the anterior pituitary
- **D.** depends on the release of hypothalamic-releasing factors into the primary capillary plexus in median eminence
- **E.** A and C are correct

588. The adrenal hormone cortisol plays a major role in
- **A.** hydrogen ion excretion
- **B.** sodium chloride retention
- **C.** maintaining blood sugar levels
- **D.** calcium excretion
- **E.** A, B, and C are correct

589. Excessive circulating levels of growth hormone are associated with
- **A.** accelerated bone maturation
- **B.** decrease in the body glycogen stores
- **C.** mobilization of fatty acids from adipose tissue
- **D.** increased concentration of amino acids in blood
- **E.** A and C are correct

590. Secretion of adrenocorticotropic hormone (ACTH)
  A. supports the adrenal medulla
  B. in excess, causes hypertrophy of the adrenal cortex
  C. does not evoke the secretion of the adrenal hormones cortisol and corticosterone
  D. is released into the anterior pituitary circulation from neurons with cell bodies in the hypothalamus
  E. B and D are correct

591. During a normal menstrual cycle
  A. the lifetime of the corpus luteum is about 30 days
  B. the rising concentration of estrogen secreted by the ripening follicle triggers the luteinizing hormone (LH) peak
  C. ovulation will occur exactly 14 days after the last vaginal bleeding
  D. the corpus luteum is controlled by the FSH concentration in the blood
  E. A and C are correct

592. Luteinizing hormone (LH) in males
  A. stimulates secretion of testosterone
  B. has a trophic effect on the Leydig cells
  C. A and B are correct
  D. acts on the seminiferous tubules to encourage sperm formation
  E. all are correct

593. Luteinizing hormone
  A. triggers ovulation
  B. supports the corpus luteum
  C. increases blood flow to the ovary
  D. causes the secretion of progesterone by the follicle, which in turn causes the release of an enzyme that breaks open the follicle
  E. all are correct

594. A large dose of exogenous insulin would result in
  A. decreased secretion of glucagon
  B. increased movement of glucose from the blood into many cells of the body
  C. increased secretion of beta cells of the pancreas
  D. decreased secretory activity of the alpha cells of the pancreas
  E. A and C are correct

595. Thyroid-stimulating hormone (TSH)
   A. promotes iodine trapping
   B. decreases thyroglobulin iodination
   C. increases the movement of thyroglobulin into follicle cells
   D. A and C are correct
   E. all are correct

596. Thyrocalcitonin
   A. is secreted by the parathyroid
   B. increases mobilization of Ca^{2+} from bone
   C. is secreted by the thyroid
   D. increases Ca^{2+} absorption by the stomach
   E. A and C are correct

597. The specific effect of thyroid hormones on the basal metabolic rate (BMR)
   A. requires the stimulation of the sodium pump by the thyroid hormones
   B. persists for several hours after the disappearance of a single dose of T_4
   C. is almost completely due to the stimulation of metabolism of skeletal muscle
   D. results in decreased oxygen consumption when thyroid hormone levels are increased
   E. all are correct

598. Oxytocin
   A. is secreted directly from nerve endings
   B. secretion is associated with neural activity
   C. is secreted by the posterior pituitary (neurohypophysis)
   D. is secreted by the anterior pituitary (adenohypophysis)
   E. A, B, and C are correct

599. The ovarian follicles
   A. secrete estrogens
   B. secrete progestins
   C. A and B are correct
   D. secrete luteinizing hormone
   E. all are correct

600. In amino acid metabolism in an adult
   A. all 20 amino acids can be completely oxidized to CO_2 and water after deamination
   B. all 20 amino acids give rise to ammonia by transamination or oxidative deamination during degradation
   C. A and B are correct
   D. all 20 amino acids are glucogenic
   E. all are correct

601. Regarding lipid metabolism
   A. chylomicrons are formed in the liver
   B. chylomicrons have a half-life of 2 hours
   C. high-density lipoproteins (HDLs) are the major source of plasma triglycerides during overnight fast
   D. low-density lipoproteins (LDLs) contain apoproteins specific for the receptor-mediated uptake of LDL by most tissues
   E. B and D are correct

602. The known hormone(s) NOT released by the islet of Langerhans is(are)
   A. pancreatic polypeptide
   B. glucagon
   C. thyroxine
   D. somatostatin
   E. A and C are correct

603. The source of insulin is
   A. alpha cells
   B. sigma cells
   C. beta cells
   D. paracrine cells
   E. none are correct

604. Insulin secretion is
   A. inhibited by fuel excess
   B. stimulated by blood glucose levels as low as 10 mg/dL
   C. inhibited by exercise
   D. stimulated by sulfonylurea compounds
   E. A and C are correct

605. Once insulin is secreted
  A. the majority is excreted via the kidneys
  B. it has a plasma half-life of 30 to 40 min
  C. it circulates bound to albumin
  D. it is degraded principally in the liver and kidney
  E. B and D are correct

606. The binding of insulin to receptor stimulates uptake of
  A. phosphate and potassium
  B. calcium
  C. glucose
  D. fatty acids
  E. A, B, and C are correct

607. Which of the following hormones is **NOT** secreted by the adeno-hypophysis?
  A. ACTH
  B. ADH
  C. Growth hormone
  D. TSH
  E. FSH

608. The hormone with the shortest half-life in the bloodstream in the following list is
  A. insulin
  B. T_3
  C. ACTH
  D. epinephrine
  E. acetylcholine

609. Urinary 17-ketosteroids
  A. are not found in women
  B. reflect the total production of androgenic substances
  C. indicate the total production of sex hormones
  D. include testosterone
  E. are highly active androgens

610. Parathyroid hormone
  A. is released when serum Ca^{2+} is too high
  B. inactivates vitamin D
  C. is secreted if serum Ca^{2+} is too low

D. works in the same direction as thyrocalcitonin
E. depends on vitamin K for adequate activity

611. The development of normal lactation depends on adequate amounts of all of the following **EXCEPT**
A. prolactin
B. T_3 and T_4
C. growth hormone
D. androgens
E. oxytocin

612. The hormone measured in urine to test for pregnancy is
A. pituitary luteinizing hormone
B. androgen
C. progesterone
D. chorionic gonadotropin
E. follicle-stimulating hormone

613. If a patient presents with a very regular 29-day menstrual cycle, ovulation should occur on day
A. 5
B. 14
C. 18
D. 20
E. 29

614. The hypothalamus is required for
A. rhythmic breathing
B. synthesis of anterior pituitary hormones
C. blood pressure homeostasis
D. perception of odor
E. homeostasis of body temperature

615. During pregnancy the maximum rate of secretion of which of the following occurs during the first trimester?
A. Chorionic gonadotropin
B. Estrogen
C. Pregnanediol
D. Oxytocin
E. Hydrocortisone

616. The secretion of testosterone by the testes
- **A.** occurs in the Sertoli cells
- **B.** is the responsibility of mature sperm cells
- **C.** is under control of the sympathetic innervation of the area
- **D.** reaches peak at about 20 years of age in the normal male
- **E.** none of the above

617. The primary stimulus for insulin secretion is increased
- **A.** epinephrine blood levels
- **B.** glucagon blood levels
- **C.** glucose blood levels
- **D.** stress
- **E.** water intake

MATCHING

DIRECTIONS (Questions 618–620): The group of questions that follow consists of a set of lettered components, followed by a list of numbered words or phrases. For each numbered word or phrase, select the **one** lettered component that is **most closely** associated with it. Each lettered component may be selected once, more than once, or not at all.

- **A.** insulin
- **B.** glucagon
- **C.** both
- **D.** neither

Encourages

618. Glycogenolysis

619. Metabolic actions of epinephrine

620. Gluconeogenesis

DIRECTIONS (Questions 621–625): The set of lettered items that follow is followed by a list of numbered words or phrases. For each numbered word or phrase select

A if the item is associated with *A* only
B if the item is associated with *B* only
C if the item is associated with both *A* and *B*
D if the item is associated with neither *A* nor *B*

    A. estrogenic substances
    B. androgenic substances
    C. both
    D. neither

621. Produced by the ovary

622. Produced by the testes

623. Produced by the adrenal cortex

624. Produced in measurable amounts throughout adult life

625. Anabolic action on muscle and bone

Endocrine Physiology

Anwers and Discussion

548. (B) The major role of insulin is to facilitate the storage of foods during a meal. A portion of this activity is an increase in the synthesis of fatty acids as a preliminary to triglyceride formation. (**Ref. 2,** pp. 306–312)

549. (A) During the second trimester of pregnancy, inhibition of ovulation and uterine enlargement are maintained by high levels of estrogen and progesterone secreted by the placenta. (**Ref. 2,** pp. 412–415)

550. (D) The major function of parathormone on the kidney is to increase the excretion of phosphate ion. (**Ref. 2,** pp. 352–361)

551. (A) The glucocorticoids increase the supply of glucose in the bloodstream through several mechanisms. The most important of these are increased gluconeogenesis, increased enzyme concentrations for glucose formation, and increased substrate by mobilizing amino acids primarily from muscle. (**Ref. 2,** pp. 338–342)

552. (C) Parathyroid hormone causes an increase in circulating levels of free Ca^{2+} by mobilizing Ca^{2+} from bone and by decreasing excretion of Ca^{2+} by the kidney. (**Ref. 2,** pp. 352–361)

553. (E) All of the factors listed in the question will raise serum cholesterol. (**Ref. 2,** p. 438)

554. (A) Estrogen antagonizes growth hormones and encourages closure of the epiphyseal plate. The deposition of subcutaneous fat and development of pubic hair also require estrogen. Low estrogen secretion does not increase Na^+ and H_2O retention. (**Ref. 2,** pp. 386–388)

555. (E) Nearly all aspects of an organism's development and maintenance, including the ones mentioned in the question, can be traced to effects associated with the endocrine system. (**Ref. 2,** p. 255)

556. (E) The relationship between hormone secretion and neural function is so intimate that the distinction between the two systems is increasingly obscured. Peptides once thought of as classic endocrine products have been found in such diverse places as the brain and neural tissue. (**Ref. 2,** p. 255)

557. (C) Neurons possess both autocrine and paracrine effects; however, by definition, the neurocrine, like the endocrine, involves transport of the hormonal signal via the circulatory system from a point of origin (secretion) in the nerve to a target cell (or tissue) some distance away. (**Ref. 2,** p. 32)

558. (C) Depending on the route of transmission, the same messenger molecule may function as a neurotransmitter only (axonal transmission), an endocrine hormone only (bloodstream), or both (transmitted both axonally and by the blood as a neurohormone), or the messenger molecule may act locally (paracrine or autocrine). (**Ref. 2,** p. 32)

559. (E) Post-transcriptional modification takes place in the nucleus. The mRNA directs synthesis of preprohormone which is then cleaved of its N-terminal to form prohormone. The final cleavage takes place in secretory granules and co-peptides are synthesized and secreted along with the hormone. (**Ref. 2,** pp. 32–34)

560. (C) Catecholamines and protein hormones are typical of a unicellular mode of hormone synthesis and release. The hormones are active at the time of release and generally need no further modification to express their activity. Stored in granules, they are modified and released by exocytosis. Another example of a unicellular mode of hormone synthesis and release is the production and release of thyroid and steroid hormones. These are simply compartmentalized during modification and are released into the cytosol and subsequently diffuse through cell membrane. (**Ref. 2,** pp. 329–331)

561. (**B**) Vitamin D, a sterol, is synthesized in the skin with very low activity which requires modification by the liver and kidneys to produce its most potent active form. Angiotensin, a peptide hormone, is synthesized from a globulin precursor released from the liver. This globulin precursor is enzymatically and sequentially modified in the kidneys and lungs. Adrenalin is typical of unicellular synthesis and release. Estrogens are produced from androgens in the gonads in a cell-to-cell sequential synthesis pathway. (**Ref. 2,** pp. 357–358)

562. (**E**) All of the factors mentioned in the question are mechanisms associated with hormonal control. Their pattern of hormonal control seems to be dictated by rhythms that may be encoded genetically, such as the patterns of hormone secretion that occur when an individual enters puberty. (**Ref. 2,** pp. 399–405)

563. (**E**) The principle of negative feedback acts to limit output of both hormone and product. In general, anything that changes the level of product serum levels will have a feedback effect on hormone secretion. For example, if a hormone is designed to increase production of product or retard its utilization, it will be inhibited by increased product serum levels. On the other hand, if the secretion of a hormone is designed to retard product production or accelerate product uptake, then the inhibitory effect is a low serum level of product. (**Ref. 2,** pp. 32–36)

564. (**C**) Steroid hormone receptor sites are located in the cytosol and the nucleus. Thyroid hormone receptors are principally in the nucleus, while peptide, protein, and catecholamine hormone receptors are located on the cell surface. These are typically polar moieties which do not cross cell membranes, unlike relatively non-polar steroid hormones. Hormone receptors are very large protein molecules present in very large numbers, perhaps to avoid problems associated with saturation kinetics. In addition, plasma membrane receptors usually contain carbohydrates and occasionally phospholipids. (**Ref. 2,** pp. 34–41)

565. (B) Since the association of a hormone with its receptor is a reversible reaction, the chemical kinetics can be expressed in terms of a K value for the association. Accordingly, this reaction follows saturation kinetics. As the concentration of free hormone increases, [H] $\rightarrow$ infinity, the concentration of bound hormone increases until it reaches receptor capacity, [HR] $\rightarrow$ receptor capacity. At this point all receptors are occupied by hormone. At the same time the ratio of bound hormone to free hormone decreases and approaches zero, [HR]/[H] $\rightarrow$ 0. The ratio of bound hormone to free hormone can be plotted as a function of bound hormone. Such plot usually yields a straight line, the slope of which equals the negative of the association constant, and the X intercept equals the receptor capacity. (**Ref. 2,** pp. 32–36)

566. (C) As long as the intracellular steps in hormone action are not rate limiting, anything that increases receptor site number or affinity increases the sensitivity of the cell. Factors affecting affinity include: pH, osmolality, and ion concentration, as well as hormone levels. Generally, receptor capacity is regulated by its own hormone. High hormone levels result in down-regulation by the cells decreasing the number of receptor sites. Conversely, low hormone levels tend to increase receptor site numbers. (**Ref. 2,** pp. 32–36)

567. (D) Lysozymal degradation of the internalized receptor-hormone complex is part of the receptor recycling system of the cell. It is unclear whether or not the internalized complex initiates any intracellular hormonal action before it is disrupted and degraded. (**Ref. 2,** pp. 34–41)

568. (C) Binding of hormone to receptor results in conformational changes in the regulatory subunit of adenylate cyclase. GTP binds to it, activating the catalytic subunit to act on Mg-ATP to form cAMP. GTP is simultaneously converted to GDP which is then less able to activate the catalytic subunit. (**Ref. 3,** pp. 38–40)

569. (C) Although intracellular concentrations of calcium ions may increase, it is the binding of the calcium ion to its binding protein calmodulin in various proportions which acts to amplify cellular enzyme and metabolic activities. The effect of the calcium-calmodulin is to regulate by activation and deactivation of enzymatic and metabolic pathways. (**Ref. 2,** pp. 35–40)

570. (A) Steroid hormones, particularly thyroid hormones, are specific for cytoplasmic receptors and induce cellular response by interacting with DNA. This is accomplished by first binding to receptor protein inside the cell. This hormone-receptor complex then enters the nucleus where it combines with acceptor proteins. This combination of hormone receptor/protein receptor interacts with chromatin containing target DNA promoter sites. This process logically explains the usually slower response elicited by steroid hormones. (**Ref. 2**, pp. 34–35)

571. (B) The binding of hormone to receptor causes the formation and release of phosphotidyl inositol-4,5-bis-phosphate. Cleavage by phospholipase A_2 and C to inositol triphosphate and diacylglycerate (DAG). DAG is cleaved to give arachidonic acid, which is a substrate for prostaglandin synthesis. (**Ref. 2**, pp. 37–40)

572. (E) Basal level of activity can be observed independent of added hormone; therefore, there is a minimal threshold of hormone concentration required to elicit a measurable response. Other features include duration of response and the effects of antagonistic or synergistic hormones. (**Ref. 2**, pp. 33–35)

573. (B) Hormonal responses are not all-or-none: a minimal concentration is required for a measurable response. The concentration of hormone required to elicit a half-measurable response defines the sensitivity of the target cell. Saturation dose defines the maximal response of the cell. Intrinsic basal level activity can be observed long after any previous exposure and independent of any added hormone. (**Ref. 2**, pp. 32–35)

574. (A) Plasma half-life is correlated with extent of protein binding. Thyroid and steroid hormones are generally protein bound which extends the half-life. In some instances, molecules may return to plasma by way of the lymphatic system. (**Ref. 2**, pp. 36–37)

575. (C) Metabolic clearance rate is defined as plasma cleared per unit time or mass hormone removed per unit time divided by the circulating mass per unit volume of plasma. MCR = mg/min removed/mg/mL of plasma = mL cleared/min. The ratio of MCR/volume of distribution of hormone = fractional turnover rate (K). (**Ref. 2**, pp. 33–35)

576. (D) Under ordinary conditions fat provides 57% of our calories. Carbohydrates provide approximately 43%. The basal metabolic requirements can be expressed in terms of the amount of CO_2 produced per milliliter of O_2 consumed. This is referred to as the respiratory quotient (RQ). Carbohydrates account for only 1% of the energy stores as compared to protein (23%) and fat (76%). (**Ref. 2,** pp. 255–258)

577. (A) The sources of glucose in overnight fasting are gluconeogenesis (25%) and glycogenolysis (75%), with 45% of glucose being used by the brain. (**Ref. 2,** pp. 261–267)

578. (E) Progesterone suppresses fertility. (**Ref. 2,** p. 379)

579. (C) Estrogens are secreted by a variety of tissues, but not by the liver. (**Ref. 2,** pp. 405–407)

580. (C) Both androgens and FSH are required for the normal development and maturation of sperm. (**Ref. 2,** pp. 391–394)

581. (E) The extension of the life of the corpus luteum for two weeks by HCG is essential for maintenance of the uterine wall during early pregnancy. The conceptus has begun to divide before it leaves the fallopian tube. Uterine engorgement is maintained by luteal progesterone. After two weeks the corpus luteum degenerates. (**Ref. 2,** pp. 412–415)

582. (C) The secretion of glucocorticosteroids is directly proportional and arranged in a negative feedback loop with the secretion of ACTH. Furthermore, these hormones will be released when CNS functions change under stress. (**Ref. 2,** pp. 342–344)

583. (E) Estrogen causes mucosal thickening with cornification of the superficial vaginal epithelium. Mitotic figures appear in the basal layer of the vaginal mucus with growth and differentiation in the intermediate and superficial layers. In addition, there is a very heavy glycogen deposition in the intermediate and superficial layers. This glycogen deposition is very important in the maintenance of the low vaginal pH (4 to 5), which protects against infection. The low pH is a result of the vaginal bacteria which acts upon the glycogen breakdown products to produce lactic acid. (**Ref. 2,** pp. 405–409)

584. (E) As a result of hyperglycemia in the diabetic, there is so much glucose in the glomerular filtrate that the transport maximum is exceeded and glucose spills into the urine. An increase in appetite compensates for urinary loss of glucose. Glucose in the filtrate also causes an osmotic hindrance to water reabsorption in the proximal and distal tubules, resulting in osmotic diuresis. Furthermore, the copious urine flow causes dehydration and stimulates thirst. Thus the diabetic is constantly thirsty and drinks large volumes of water. **(Ref. 2,** pp. 312–316)

585. (A) Pituitary hormone secretion has a negative feedback relationship to many of its target organs. This means that if the target organ secretions are low, pituitary trophic secretions will be high. **(Ref. 2,** pp. 365–368)

586. (B) The hormones of the thyroid do not have any discrete target organ or systems and their effects are diffuse, being manifest throughout the body. Their effects are observed after a considerable lag or latency that may last for several days, indicating that these hormones appear to play a role in long-term functions rather than instant minute-to-minute regulation. Furthermore, these hormones appear to not be essential for maintaining life, albeit their lack certainly reduces the quality of life. **(Ref. 2,** pp. 290–300)

587. (D) Adenohypophyseal secretions are stimulated by releasing factors formed in hypothalamic neurons and released into the primary capillary plexus in the median eminence. **(Ref. 2,** pp. 365–367)

588. (E) The adrenal cortex behaves as two different endocrine glands. It secretes the mineralocorticoid aldosterone which enhances excretion of sodium and hydrogen while retaining potassium. The cortex also secretes cortisol which helps to sustain blood sugar and blood pressure. **(Ref. 2,** pp. 332–336)

589. (C) Overproduction of growth hormones will result in a prominent increase in bone growth with delayed maturation. In addition, growth hormone will favor protein production over all other biochemical paths and, hence, a mobilization of fatty acids from adipose tissue for energy. **(Ref. 2,** pp. 368–376)

590. **(A)** ACTH will cause the secretion of cortisol and corticosterone from the adrenal cortex after its release from cells in the anterior pituitary. (**Ref. 2,** pp. 332–336)

591. **(B)** During a normal menstrual cycle the rising concentration of estrogen secreted by the ripening follicle triggers the LH peak, which causes ovulation. In the case where fertilization does not occur, the lifetime of the corpus luteum is about 10 days. (**Ref. 2,** pp. 399–405)

592. **(C)** The major role of luteinizing hormone in the male is the support of the Leydig cells and stimulation of testosterone secretion. However, LH is also needed to induce the Leydig cells to make the testosterone needed for spermatogenesis. (**Ref. 2,** pp. 391–393)

593. **(E)** Luteinizing hormone supports the ovary by increasing blood flow to that organ. In addition, this hormone triggers ovulation by increasing progesterone secretion, which in turn causes the release of an enzyme that breaks open the follicle. After ovulation, LH supports the continued existence of the ovum. (**Ref. 2,** pp. 399–404)

594. **(B)** A large dose of exogenous insulin would lower blood glucose levels by encouraging the movement of glucose into most of the cells of the body. This lowered glucose level would cause a reflex increased secretion of glucagon. (**Ref. 2,** pp. 316–323)

595. **(D)** Thyroid-stimulating hormone promotes iodine trapping, increases the movement of thyroglobulin, and increases thyroglobulin iodination. (**Ref. 2,** pp. 299–300)

596. **(C)** Thyrocalcitonin is secreted by the thyroid gland and is important in control of Ca^{2+} mobilization from bone. (**Ref. 2,** pp. 352–353, 359–364)

597. **(A)** The effect of thyroid hormones on the basal metabolic rate persists for several days after a single dose of T_4 and is blocked by ovulation. (**Ref. 2,** pp. 296–298)

598. **(E)** Oxytocin is a hormone that is secreted from nerve endings found in the posterior pituitary gland. (**Ref. 1,** pp. 365–366)

599. (C) The ovarian follicles supply both of the major classes of ovarian hormones (estrogens and progestins) in addition to supplying the gametes for reproduction. (**Ref. 2,** pp. 405–411)

600. (C) Leucine is the only amino acid that is not glucogenic. (**Ref. 2,** pp. 268–270)

601. (D) Chylomicrons are formed from dietary fat and are absorbed through the intestine. They have a half-life of 5 min. They are rapidly acted upon by lipoprotein lipase to liberate free fatty acids in adipose, heart, and muscle tissue. Chylomicron remnants give rise to LDL and bile salts in the liver. (**Ref. 2,** pp. 277–280)

602. (C) In addition to somatostatin and pancreatic polypeptide, insulin and glucagon are released by the islet of Langerhans. (**Ref. 2,** pp. 306–312)

603. (C) Insulin: beta cells; glucagon: alpha cells; somatostatin: sigma cells. (**Ref. 2,** pp. 306–308)

604. (B) Some stimulators besides carbohydrates include: protein, free fatty acids, ketoacids, glucagon, potassium, calcium, and sulfonylurea drugs. Inhibitors include: fasting, exercise, somatostatin, prostaglandins, and drugs such as diazoxide and phenytoin. (**Ref. 2,** pp. 317–320)

605. (E) Very little insulin is excreted unchanged into the urine. It circulates unbound to any carrier proteins. As a result, insulin has a very short half-life, 5 to 8 min. Degradation takes place principally in the liver and kidneys. (**Ref. 2,** pp. 306–312)

606. (A) Insulin stimulates cellular uptake of amino acids as well as certain ions such as magnesium, potassium, and phosphate. (**Ref. 2,** pp. 308–312)

607. (B) Antidiuretic hormone (ADH) is secreted by the posterior pituitary. (**Ref. 2,** pp. 365–374)

608. (E) Because of powerful esterases in the blood, acetylcholine has an extremely short half-life. (**Ref. 2,** pp. 87–89)

609. (B) Both androsterone and dehydroepiandrosterone are 17-keto-steroids. These are excreted either into the gut in the bile or into the urine. The rate of excretion of 17-ketosteroids in the urine is an index of the rate of androgen production in the body. **(Ref. 2,** pp. 405–409)

610. (C) Parathyroid hormone attempts to raise serum calcium if it falls below normal. **(Ref. 2,** pp. 359–361)

611. (D) Androgens are not significant for the development of lactation. **(Ref. 2,** pp. 415–417)

612. (D) Chorionic gonadotropin rises precipitously during the first trimester of pregnancy. **(Ref. 2,** pp. 413–414)

613. (B) Ovulation occurs regularly 14 days before the onset of menstruation. **(Ref. 2,** pp. 399–406)

614. (E) Large areas of the anterior hypothalamus, especially the preoptic area, are concerned with regulation of body temperature. **(Ref. 2,** pp. 227–232)

615. (A) Coincidentally with the development of the trophoblast, cells from early fertilized ovum, the hormone chorionic gonadotropin is secreted by the syncytial trophoblastic cells into the fluid of the mother. The rate of secretion rises rapidly to reach a maximum approximately 7 weeks after ovulation and decreases to a relatively low value 16 weeks after ovulation. Without this secretion the uterus (with its implanted ovum) would slough off. **(Ref. 2,** pp. 412–415)

616. (D) Testosterone is secreted from the cells of Leydig and reaches peak levels in the late teens and early twenties. **(Ref. 2,** pp. 341–345)

617. (C) The primary stimulus for insulin secretion is an increase in blood glucose levels. **(Ref. 2,** pp. 306–312)

618. (B) Glucagon stimulates the breakdown of glycogen. **(Ref. 2,** pp. 320–322)

619. (B) Glucagon and epinephrine are additive in many of the metabolic effects. (**Ref. 2,** pp. 320–322)

620. (B) Glucagon has a significant effect on increasing blood glucose even after all the glycogen in the liver has been exhausted. This results from increasing the rate of gluconeogenesis in the liver cells by increasing extraction of amino acids from the blood, which are then converted to glucose. (**Ref. 2,** pp. 320–322)

621. (C) In normal, non-pregnant females both estrogens and androgens are secreted by the ovaries but only estrogens are exclusively secreted in major quantities only by the ovaries. (**Ref. 2,** pp. 399–408)

622. (C) In addition to testosterone, small amounts of estrogens are found in the male testes. (**Ref. 2,** pp. 391–395)

623. (B) The adrenal cortex secretes at least five different androgens. (**Ref. 2,** pp. 338–339)

624. (C) Testosterone production increases rapidly at the onset of puberty and lasts throughout the remainder of life. At puberty estrogens increase twentyfold. Estrogens are produced in subcritical quantities for a short time after menopause. (**Ref. 2,** pp. 395–398)

625. (C) One of the most important male characteristics is the development of increasing musculature following puberty. The bones grow considerably in thickness and also deposit considerable calcium salts. Estrogens cause increased osteoblastic activity and also a slight increase in total body protein. (**Ref. 2,** pp. 386–388)

8

Gastrointestinal Physiology

MULTIPLE CHOICE

DIRECTIONS (Questions 626–692): Each of the questions or incomplete statements below is followed by five suggested answers or completions. Select the **one** that is **best** in each case.

626. The sugars normally found in significant amounts in the intestinal chyme include
- **A.** glucose and fructose
- **B.** galactose and xylose
- **C.** mannose and ribose
- **D.** mannose and xylose
- **E.** ribose and xylose

627. Man is unable to digest dietary
- **A.** glycogen
- **B.** dextrin
- **C.** saccharose
- **D.** cellulose
- **E.** glucose

628. Specific dynamic action is
- **A.** the specific effects of pharmacologic agents on the gastrointestinal tract
- **B.** the effect of certain foodstuffs on metabolic rate
- **C.** the effect of parasympathetic stimulation on metabolic rate
- **D.** the effect of sympathetic stimulation on metabolic rate
- **E.** the effect of exercise on metabolic rate

629. Gastric secretion is
- **A.** increased by stomach distension
- **B.** stimulated by an increase in phonic activity
- **C.** stimulated by norepinephrine
- **D.** inhibited by curare
- **E.** not affected by the presence of food in the stomach

630. Which of the following is **NOT** associated with pancreatic secretions?
- **A.** Source of HCO_3^- for the neutralization of gastric acid in the small intestine
- **B.** Contains most of the digestive enzymes
- **C.** Reduces the osmolality of the fluid in the gut
- **D.** Source of tributyrase
- **E.** Has a pH that is primarily controlled by ventilation of the lungs

631. Primary peristalsis and secondary peristalsis of the esophagus are different in that the latter
- **A.** is more rapid
- **B.** is independent of neural control
- **C.** is initiated by swallowing
- **D.** is confined to the upper esophagus
- **E.** is under intrinsic neuronal control

632. Which of the following is **NOT** associated with the motor function of the stomach?
- **A.** storage
- **B.** mixing
- **C.** chyme formation
- **D.** rapid emptying to accommodate entry of excess food into the stomach
- **E.** none of the above are associated with the motor function of the stomach

633. In Figure 27, the major pathway(s) for water movement from the mucosal side to the serosal side of the intestinal mucosa is(are) indicated by which arrows?
   A. 1, 2, and 3
   B. 1 and 3
   C. 2 and 4
   D. 4 only
   E. All of the above

634. The secretion of intrinsic factor occurs in the
   A. parietal cells of the stomach
   B. chief cells of the stomach
   C. upper duodenum
   D. beta cells of the pancreas
   E. liver

635. Ingested cholesterol enters the intestinal epithelial cell by
   A. diffusion through the lipid portion of the cell membrane
   B. diffusion through pores in the cell membrane
   C. an active transport mechanism
   D. pinocytosis
   E. esterification, diffusion through pores, and then hydrolysis

Figure 27

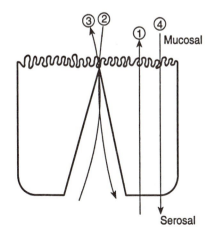

636. Vitamin D is essential for normal
   A. glucose absorption
   B. fat absorption
   C. protein absorption
   D. Ca^{2+} absorption
   E. antidiuretic hormone (ADH) secretion

637. Salivary secretion
   A. has a constant composition regardless of the rate of secretion
   B. is probably a simple ultrafiltrate of plasma
   C. has the same constituency no matter what kind of material is placed in the mouth
   D. is entirely under neural control
   E. is entirely under cortical control

638. The pacemaker for small intestine motility
   A. lies in the fundal region of the stomach
   B. controls the motility of all of the small intestine
   C. only controls a small area of gut near the bile duct
   D. lies in the radial muscle of the gut near the pyloric sphincter
   E. lies in the cerebrum (pacemaker cells are not present in the GI system)

639. Distension of the stomach
   A. is associated with a decrease in peristaltic activity in the stomach
   B. decreases tone of the lower esophageal sphincter
   C. causes an acute increase in pressure inside the resting stomach
   D. results in a potentially large increase in volume with very little pressure change
   E. is under cerebral control, as it is solely influenced by psychic factors

640. Secretin is released by
   A. acid in the duodenum
   B. acid in the urine
   C. S cells in the duodenal mucosa
   D. distention of the colon
   E. cells in the hypothalamus

641. The secretion of bile from the liver
   A. is not necessary for normal digestion
   B. contains large amounts of high-protein solution
   C. is important only for the normal digestion of proteins
   D. is stored in the gallbladder
   E. is important only for the normal digestion of sugars

642. Amino acid absorption
   A. is linked to Na^+
   B. is not stereospecific
   C. depends on glucose being present in the duodenal lumen
   D. depends on the Ca^{2+} concentration in the duodenal lumen
   E. A and C are correct

643. When an obese but otherwise normal person goes on a diet limited in calories
   A. initial weight loss exceeds initial fat loss
   B. body fat is lost at a rate proportionate to the caloric deficiency of the diet
   C. initial weight loss is due primarily to water loss
   D. body water is lost at an increased rate
   E. B and D are correct

644. The symptoms associated with the congenital absence of lactase
   A. is most frequently observed in infants
   B. is characterized by an intolerance of milk
   C. results in diarrhea following ingestion of lactose
   D. may be present in a person who tolerates sucrose and maltose
   E. all are correct

645. Gastric secretion normally occurs in response to
   A. duodenal distension
   B. emotional disturbance
   C. gastrin release
   D. sight and smell of food
   E. A and C are correct

646. Secretions of the small intestinal mucosa
   A. are stimulated by gastrin
   B. contain all of the enzymes necessary for digestion
   C. contain disaccharidases that are very important for normal carbohydrate digestion
   D. serve primarily a protective function
   E. B and D are correct

647. After free fatty acids and glycerol enter the epithelial cells, these compounds
   A. are resynthesized into triglycerides
   B. move out of the cell by simple diffusion
   C. are mostly carried away by the bloodstream
   D. are transported out of the cell by specific carrier systems
   E. A and C are correct

648. Which of the following is associated with oxyntic gland secretion
   A. mucus
   B. pepsinogen
   C. intrinsic factor
   D. hydrochloric acid
   E. all of the above

649. Lipid absorption
   A. is facilitated by specific transport proteins in the brush border
   B. is accelerated by the formation of micelles
   C. depends on the lipid solubility of lipase for hydrolysis of triglycerides
   D. is facilitated by pancreatic enzymes
   E. B and D are correct

650. Bile salts
   A. are not reabsorbed
   B. are absorbed in the stomach
   C. are absorbed chiefly in the ileum
   D. are absorbed in the duodenum
   E. A and C are correct

651. Sodium transport in the gastrointestinal system
  A. may include calcium or magnesium exchange
  B. depends on sodium ion carriers found on the basal and lateral borders of the epithelial cells in the duodenum
  C. is a passive process as it leaves the epithelial cells of the duodenum
  D. is down an electrochemical gradient as it enters the epithelial cells of the duodenum
  E. B and D are correct

652. Glucose
  A. is linked to sodium ion absorption
  B. requires no energy to remove sodium ion from the epithelial cell
  C. probably depends on a carrier that requires both sodium ion and glucose for movement of the sugar into the epithelial cell
  D. requires energy for the movement of glucose into the epithelial cell
  E. A and C are correct

653. Secretin
  A. is secreted by the pancreas
  B. increases pancreatic secretion of HCO_3^-
  C. stimulates pancreatic secretion of lysine
  D. is released from the mucosa of the large intestine
  E. B and D are correct

654. Vitamin B_{12} absorption
  A. depends on the presence of intrinsic factor
  B. depends on passive diffusion
  C. occurs in the jujenum
  D. occurs in the stomach
  E. A and C are correct

655. The movement of lipid out of the epithelial cells
  A. depends on the lymph system
  B. is abnormal in a beta-lipoprotein
  C. depends on the formation of chylomicra
  D. depends on packaging of the lipid in a protein envelope
  E. all are correct

656. Lipid absorption
- **A.** is Na⁺ linked
- **B.** requires formation of chylomicra
- **C.** depends on liver bile for a normal time course
- **D.** is by active transport through the brush border
- **E.** A and C are correct

657. Absorption of materials from the gastrointestinal tract
- **A.** is facilitated by the increase in surface area provided by the physical arrangement of the small intestine
- **B.** cannot occur against an electrochemical energy gradient
- **C.** will depend on the ability of compounds with molecular weights over 180 to diffuse through a lipid barrier unless a specific transport system is available
- **D.** depends on the active pumping of water
- **E.** A and C are correct

658. Motility of the small intestine is stimulated by
- **A.** gastrin
- **B.** cholecystokinin
- **C.** A and B are correct
- **D.** acetylcholine (ACh)
- **E.** all are correct

659. The act of swallowing is associated with
- **A.** concurrent inhibition of respiration
- **B.** opening of the glottis
- **C.** movement of food into the nasopharynx
- **D.** upper esophageal sphincter constriction when food is placed in contact with the anterior pillars of the pharynx
- **E.** A and C are correct

660. Amino acid absorption
- **A.** may require energy to remove sodium ions from epithelial cells
- **B.** may not require energy for movement of amino acid into epithelial cells
- **C.** may be mediated through a carrier that requires amino acid and sodium ion for activation
- **D.** may use the concentration gradient of sodium ions from the gut lumen to the epithelial intracellular compartment to sup-

ply the energy for amino acid movement out of the gut and into the epithelial cells

E. all of the above

661. Calcium absorption is enhanced by
   A. high-fat, low-protein diet
   B. elevated phosphate intake
   C. vitamin D in the diet
   D. raising the pH of the intestinal contents
   E. B and D are correct

662. The effect of increased vagal stimulation on the intestine is
   A. decreased oxygen consumption
   B. decreased rate of muscle spike potentials
   C. hyperpolarization of smooth muscle membrane
   D. increased motility
   E. B and D are correct

663. Which of the following is associated with the esophageal phase of swallowing?
   A. Sealing off of the nasopharynx
   B. Constriction of the upper esophageal sphincter
   C. Initiation of the secondary phase of peristalsis
   D. Begins when food bolus comes into contact with back of tongue
   E. A and C are correct

664. The presentation of a bolus of solid food to the mouth
   A. stimulates taste buds
   B. is usually followed by mastication
   C. reflexively stimulates the salivary glands
   D. results in muscular activities that are under conscious control
   E. all are correct

665. The gallbladder
   A. can be caused to contract by cholecystokinin
   B. can be caused to contract by vagal activity
   C. A and B are correct
   D. is stimulated to contract by activity in certain sympathetic nerves
   E. all are correct

666. Gastric peristalsis
   A. originates in the distal half of the stomach
   B. is characterized by strong contractions of the antrum at the end of the wave
   C. ejects all the contents of the antrum into the duodenum
   D. decreases in intensity as it sweeps toward the pylorus
   E. B and D are correct

667. Motility of the small intestine is
   A. inhibited by the vagus nerve
   B. stimulated by adrenergic agents
   C. totally independent of activity of the stomach
   D. stimulated by radial stretch of the gut
   E. B and D are correct

668. Deglutition (swallowing)
   A. is a complicated act requiring the precise coordination of many muscle groups
   B. is an automatic function of smooth muscle
   C. is associated with a lowering of the hard palate to prevent reflux of food into the nasopharynx
   D. does not require relaxation of cricopharyngeal muscle
   E. A and C are correct

669. Esophageal peristalsis
   A. is stimulated by ACh
   B. is initiated by vagal reflexes
   C. can be caused by distension of the esophagus
   D. is characterized by activity proximal to the pharynx inhibiting activity distal to the pharynx
   E. all are correct

670. Defecation
   A. cannot be delayed by conscious contraction of the external sphincter and levator ani muscles
   B. requires intact sympathetic innervation of the rectum for proper reflex integration
   C. depends on information from stretch receptors in the wall of the duodenum
   D. is a reflex interruption of anal continence
   E. all are correct

671. Liver bile
  A. flow from the liver is best stimulated by the presentation of increased amounts of bile to liver cells
  B. cannot be secreted against a pressure greater than aortic blood pressure
  C. formation requires anaerobic metabolism
  D. is secreted by a few select hepatic cells
  E. A and C are correct

672. Carbohydrate absorption
  A. does not require energy
  B. is not the same for fructose and glucose
  C. proceeds mainly with polysaccharides
  D. depends on diffusion of glucose through the epithelial cell membranes
  E. B and D are correct

673. Secretin
  A. is released from the gastric mucosa
  B. primarily stimulates enzyme secretion of the pancreas
  C. A and B are correct
  D. stimulates bicarbonate and fluid secretions by the pancreas
  E. all are correct

674. Cholecystokinin
  A. release is stimulated by protein hydrolysates in the lumen of the small intestine
  B. is released from gastric mucosa cells
  C. has no structural relationship to gastrin
  D. release is stimulated by distension of the colon
  E. A and C are correct

675. Liver bile flow is increased by
  A. gastrin
  B. pancreatic secretion
  C. vagal stimulation
  D. sympathetic nerve stimulation
  E. A and C are correct

676. Gastrin
  A. decreases HCl secretion
  B. is released by ethanol in the stomach
  C. is released by sympathetic stimulation
  D. is released by stomach emptying
  E. B and D are correct

677. Motility of the colon is
  A. stimulated by acetylcholine
  B. stimulated by norepinephrine
  C. primarily inhibited by the vagus nerve
  D. stimulated by distension of the ileum
  E. A and C are correct

678. Salivary secretion
  A. has a serous component
  B. has a mucous component
  C. A and B are correct
  D. is largely under hormonal control
  E. all are correct

679. Hydrochloric acid secretion
  A. is accomplished by passive diffusion
  B. requires the dissociation of water with subsequent exchange of the hydrogen ion for potassium ion
  C. requires anaerobic metabolism
  D. utilizes protein molecules to neutralize OH_ remaining in the secretory cell
  E. B and D are correct

680. The chyme entering the small intestine causes a release of secretin which results in
  A. stimulation of pancreatic fluid in which there are no enzymes
  B. a pancreatic fluid that aids in protection against the development of duodenal ulcers
  C. a pancreatic secretion whose pH is just right for action of the pancreatic enzymes that are eventually released
  D. pancreatic fluid secretion of a large volume containing low chloride but high bicarbonate concentration
  E. all are correct

681. The rate of gastric emptying is
   A. primarily controlled by the glucose concentration in the saliva
   B. affected by the resistance to flow offered by the pylorus
   C. increased by the presence of fats, acid, or protein hydrolysates in the duodenum
   D. unrelated to the volume introduced into the stomach
   E. B and D are correct

682. Vomiting
   A. results in dehydration, depletion of a body HCO_3^-, Na^+ and K^+, and alkalosis
   B. is the forceful expulsion of the contents of the digestive tract through the mouth
   C. results in loss of fluid, and if prolonged, can result in circulatory collapse and death
   D. is a complex reflex act, which is coordinated by a center located in the sacral region of the spinal cord
   E. A, B, and C are correct

683. Oxyntic or parietal cells secrete
   A. HCl
   B. trypsin
   C. zymogen granules
   D. pepsinogen
   E. A and C are correct

684. The stomach is a poor area for absorption primarily because
   A. most foods are swallowed before ptyalin has a chance to break down starch
   B. pH of the stomach is too high
   C. the junction between epithelial cells presents wide spaces for fluid/ion movement
   D. the stomach lacks villus membranes
   E. B and D are correct

685. Absorption of water through the intestinal membrane
   A. follows usual laws of osmosis
   B. may be transported from plasma into chyme
   C. A and B are correct
   D. occurs when the chyme is concentrated
   E. all are correct

686. In carbohydrate absorption
- **A.** transport is non-selective
- **B.** it is highest for glucose
- **C.** carbohydrates are absorbed almost entirely as disaccharides
- **D.** carbohydrates display competitive absorption
- **E.** all are correct

687. Various secretions along the alimentary tract
- **A.** provide protection of the mucosa
- **B.** serve as lubrication to aid in digestion
- **C.** are formed in response to ingestion of food
- **D.** are regulated according to the amount of food consumed
- **E.** all are correct

688. Stimulation of the gastrointestinal secretions includes
- **A.** chemical stimuli
- **B.** tactile stimulation
- **C.** A and B are correct
- **D.** distension
- **E.** all are correct

689. The pangs associated with hunger
- **A.** are decreased by a low level of blood sugar
- **B.** are accompanied with feelings of hunger and pain in the pit of the stomach
- **C.** usually appear 3 to 4 hours after fasting begins
- **D.** diminish after 1 to 2 days of starvation
- **E.** B and D are correct

690. Swallowing is dependent upon
- **A.** pyramidal tract
- **B.** vagus nerve
- **C.** trigeminal nerve
- **D.** seventh cranial nerves
- **E.** B and D are correct

691. The musculature of the esophagus below the pharyngeal junction is
- **A.** smooth only in lower third
- **B.** is striated in the upper third
- **C.** mixed smooth and striated muscle in the middle third

D. innervated primarily from vagal and glossopharyngeal nerves
E. all are correct

692. Enzymes associated with protein digestion coming from the stomach include
   A. pepsin
   B. trypsin
   C. carboxypolypeptidase
   D. chymotrypsin
   E. A and C are correct

MATCHING

DIRECTIONS (Questions 693–696): The group of questions that follow consists of a set of lettered components followed by a list of numbered words or phrases. For each numbered word or phrase, select the **one** lettered component that is **most closely** associated with it. Each lettered component may be selected once, more than once, or not at all

   A. protein decarboxylase
   B. vitamin A
   C. pantothenic acid
   D. folinic acid
   E. riboflavin

693. Required with thiamine in decarboxylation of pyruvic acid

694. Required as part of the co-enzyme A molecule

695. Definite nutritional requirement

696. Required for incorporation into hydrogen carrier co-enzymes

DIRECTIONS (Questions 697–700): The set of lettered items that follow is followed by a list of numbered words or phrases. For **each** numbered word or phrase **select**

A if the item is associated with *A* only
B if the item is associated with *B* only
C if the item is associated with both *A* and *B*
D if the item is associated with neither *A* nor *B*

A. sympathetic activity
B. parasympathetic activity
C. both
D. neither

697. Required for gastric phase of digestion

698. Required for cephalic phase of digestion

699. Required for mucous secretion of the large intestine

700. Involved in mucous secretion of the salivary glands

Gastrointestinal Physiology

Answers and Discussion

626. (A) Glucose and fructose are the results of sucrose hydrolysis and are very prominent in intestinal chyme. **(Ref. 2,** pp. 431–435)

627. (D) Man is unable to digest dietary cellulose, because there are no enzymes in the human alimentary tract capable of digesting it. **(Ref. 2,** pp. 431–435)

628. (B) Specific dynamic action is the ability of certain amino acids derived from protein foods to generate more heat than their caloric value. **(Ref. 2,** pp. 268–270)

629. (A) Gastric secretion is stimulated by stomach distension, vagal activity, and acetylcholine. **(Ref. 2,** pp. 450–456)

630. (A) Pancreatic juice has several important actions: It neutralizes the acidic chyme from the stomach, reduces the osmolality of fluid from the gut, and contains most of the major digestive enzymes. Tributyrase, or gastric lipase, is secreted in the stomach and is associated with triglyceride digestion. **(Ref. 2,** pp. 456–458)

631. (E) Secondary peristalsis is a local response to distension of the esophagus, while primary peristalsis is initiated by swallowing. Esophageal peristalsis functions to propel food the full length of the esophagus and is under neuronal control. However, secondary peristalsis is under enteric neuronal control. **(Ref. 2,** pp. 456–458)

632. **(D)** Storage and mixing with subsequent chyme formation is followed by slow expulsion. (**Ref. 2,** pp. 453–456)

633. **(C)** Water is absorbed from the lumen of the gut both transcellularly and across the "tight junction" between cells. (**Ref. 2,** pp. 463–466)

634. **(A)** Intrinsic factor for the absorption of vitamin B_2 is secreted by the parietal cells of the stomach. (**Ref. 2,** pp. 455–456)

635. **(A)** Cholesterol depends of its lipid solubility to diffuse through the cell membrane. (**Ref. 2,** pp. 463–467)

636. **(D)** Vitamin D is necessary for the movement of Ca^{2+} out of the gut lumen into the epithelial cells and out of the epithelial cells into circulation. (**Ref. 2,** pp. 463–465)

637. **(D)** Salivary secretion depends entirely on neural control mechanisms, mainly parasympathetic. The salivatory nuclei (in medulla and pons) are activated by tasting and tactile stimulation from the tongue and mouth. (**Ref. 2,** pp. 448–450)

638. **(B)** The pacemaker for small intestine motility lies in the longitudinal muscle coat near the bile duct. This pacemaker may dictate activity to all of the small intestine. (**Ref. 2,** pp. 463–465)

639. **(D)** As material enters the stomach, the muscle in the walls will relax to allow a relatively large change in volume with a small pressure change. Part of this relaxation process is due to the property of plasticity inherent in visceral smooth muscle (stress relaxation). (**Ref. 2,** pp. 450–455)

640. **(C)** Secretin is released by cells in the intestinal mucosa (the "S" cells) in response to acid in the duodenum. (**Ref. 2,** pp. 446–448)

641. **(D)** Liver bile, which contains lecithin and cholesterol, is secreted continuously and stored in the gallbladder for periodic release to the gut lumen. (**Ref. 2,** pp. 458–463)

642. **(A)** Amino acid absorption in the gut is stereospecific, is linked to sodium movement, and does not require glucose. (**Ref. 2,** pp. 463–466, 435–436)

643. (B) When an obese individual starts a calorie-limited diet, fat is utilized immediately to make up for the missing calories. There is also a retention of body fluid. **(Ref. 2,** pp. 284–286)

644. (E) Infants with congenital absence of lactase frequently have a watery diarrhea, but these same infants may tolerate sucrose and maltose perfectly well. **(Ref. 2,** pp. 433–434)

645. (C) Gastrin does not require an intact reflex pathway to elicit increased gastric secretion. **(Ref. 2,** pp. 450–451)

646. (D) The major secretions of the small intestine are mucous secretions for the protection of the intestinal lining. **(Ref. 2,** pp. 463–466)

647. (A) After free fatty acids and glycerol enter the epithelial cells of the gut they are re-esterified to form triglycerides before they leave the intracellular pool. **(Ref. 2,** pp. 436–438)

648. (E) Mucus, hydrochloric acid, intrinsic factor, and pepsinogen are secretions associated with the oxyntic gland found in the stomach. **(Ref. 2,** pp. 450–451)

649. (B) The formation of micellar aggregates by liver bile is crucial for the normal absorption of lipids. **(Ref. 1,** p. 788 ff)

650. (C) Bile salts are largely absorbed by an active transport system in the ileum. **(Ref. 2,** pp. 458–463)

651. (E) Sodium ion transport is down an electrochemical gradient as it enters cells of the gut but requires active transport to leave the cells of the gut. The active transport is found on the basal and lateral borders of the epithelial cells in the duodenum and is stimulated by glucose. **(Ref. 2,** pp. 463–466)

652. (E) Glucose absorption uses the normal extracellular/intracellular sodium ion gradient to assist the movement of the sugar into the epithelial cells of the gut. The sodium ion must then be removed by an energy utilizing Na^+/K^+ ATPase. **(Ref. 2,** pp. 432–435)

653. (B) The hormone secretin is secreted by the mucosa of the small intestine. It causes increases in fluid and bicarbonate secretion by the pancreas. **(Ref. 2,** pp. 446–447)

654. (A) The absorption of vitamin B_2 by the ileum requires intrinsic factor from the stomach. (**Ref. 2,** pp. 463–466)

655. (E) Once lipid material has moved into epithelial cells of the gut it is packaged in protein envelopes to form chylomicra, which are then dumped into the lymphatic system. In a beta-lipoproteinemia, this system is interrupted because adequate envelope protein is not available for producing chylomicra. (**Ref. 2,** pp. 436–438)

656. (C) Liver bile assists the diffusion of lipid digestive products across the brush border of the ileum by emulsifying the fats to increase their surface area. (**Ref. 2,** pp. 436–438)

657. (E) Absorption from the lumen of the gut is limited by the lipid solubility of compounds with molecular weights over 180 and can occur against an electrochemical energy gradient in cases of active transport. To facilitate this absorption, the gut is folded to increase the surface area available for movement of materials. (**Ref. 2,** pp. 463–466)

658. (E) Motility of the ileum is stimulated by gastrin, cholecystokinin-pancreozymin, and by ACh released from parasympathetic innervation. (**Ref. 2,** pp. 465–466)

659. (A) When swallowing occurs, the shift from the more common movement of air in and out of the lungs to the movement of solids or liquids into the stomach requires inhibition of respiration, closure of the glottis, and relaxation of the upper esophageal sphincter. (**Ref. 2,** pp. 448–450)

660. (E) Amino acid absorption uses the sodium ion gradient from the lumen into the intracellular fluid of the gut epithelium to drive amino acid transport. The sodium then must be removed from the epithelial cells by active transport. (**Ref. 2,** pp. 435–436)

661. (C) A low intestinal pH tends to keep calcium in solution and, thus, favors absorption. Vitamin D enhances the absorption of Ca^{2+} from the gut. (**Ref. 2,** p. 440)

662. (D) Increased vagal stimulation depolarizes smooth muscle cells. (**Ref. 2,** pp. 442–443)

663. **(A)** Relaxation of the upper esophageal sphincter with the subsequent initiation of the primary wave of peristalsis is associated with phase III or the esophageal phase. **(Ref. 2,** pp. 448–450)

664. **(E)** When a bolus of food is presented to the mouth, voluntary activities of mastication ensue with taste bud activation and reflex stimulation of the salivary glands. **(Ref. 2,** p. 448–450)

665. **(C)** The gallbladder is the primary storage site of liver bile and can be stimulated to contract by cholecystokinin and vagal activity. Sympathetic activity can be antagonistic. **(Ref. 2,** pp. 458–460)

666. **(B)** Gastric peristalsis is a wave of muscular contraction which starts in the fundus of the stomach and sweeps toward the antrum with a constantly increasing force of contraction. **(Ref. 2,** pp. 450–455)

667. **(D)** The primary intrinsic stimulus for the contraction of the smooth muscle of the ileum is radial stretch. **(Ref. 2,** pp. 463–466)

668. **(A)** Deglutition is a complicated act requiring precise coordination of many structures. A small portion of this activity is the raising of the soft palate to prevent reflux of food into the nasopharynx. **(Ref. 2,** p. 450)

669. **(E)** Esophageal peristalsis is a wave of muscular contraction along the esophagus that closes the lower esophageal sphincter, can be stimulated by radial stretch of the esophagus, is stimulated by ACh, and is characterized by activity proximal to the pharynx inhibiting activity distal to the pharynx. **(Ref. 2,** pp. 448–450)

670. **(D)** Defecation is a reflex activity involving stretch receptors in the rectum and the parasympathetic nervous system in a reflex arc. This reflex can be overcome by the conscious contraction of the external sphincter. **(Ref. 2,** pp. 466–470)

671. **(A)** Liver bile formation is an active process requiring energy. This energy is evident when it is noted that bile can be secreted against a pressure greater than aortic blood pressure. One of the best stimulants for bile secretion is the presentation of small

amounts of bile to the blood perfusing the liver. (**Ref. 2,** pp. 458–460)

672. **(B)** Carbohydrate absorption is an active carrier-mediated process which acts only on monosaccharides. The carriers for fructose and glucose appear to be separate systems. (**Ref. 2,** pp. 434–435)

673. **(D)** The major action of the hormone secretin is to stimulate bicarbonate and fluid secretions by the pancreas. (**Ref. 2,** pp. 443–448)

674. **(A)** The release of pancreozymin (now called cholecystokinin) from intestinal mucosa cells is stimulated by distension of the stomach and the presence of protein hydrolysates in the lumen of the small intestine. The amino acid sequence of gastrin and pancreozymin do have some elements in common. (**Ref. 2,** pp. 446–447)

675. **(C)** Secretin and vagal stimulation can increase the flow of liver bile. (**Ref. 2,** pp. 446–447)

676. **(B)** The major function of gastrin is to stimulate the secretion of HCl into the stomach as a response to food being presented to the upper GI tract. The release of gastrin can be stimulated by ethanol in the stomach, stomach distension, and vagal stimulation. (**Ref. 2,** pp. 445–446)

677. **(A)** Motility of the colon is controlled by a dual system of innervation which contains cholinergic nerves that excite and adrenergic nerves that inhibit the colon. (**Ref. 2,** pp. 466–470)

678. **(C)** Salivary secretions have both a mucous and serous component and are obtained from the carotid, submaxillary, and sublingual glands. The control of these secretions is entirely integrated by the CNS. (**Ref. 2,** pp. 448–450)

679. **(B)** The secretion of HCl by the gastric mucosa is an active energy-dependent process. It involves the dissociation into H^+ and OH^-, with active secretion of H^+ in exchange for K^+ and will combine with the actively secreted Cl^- in the canaliculus. (**Ref. 2,** pp. 450–453)

680. (E) Pancreatic secretion is humorally regulated by the hormones secretin and cholecystokinin. The chyme (which contains HCl) causes the small intestine to release and activate the hormone secretin which acts on the pancreas to release a large volume of fluid. The fluid contains a high concentration of bicarbonate (145 mEq/L) but a low concentration of chloride ion. This fluid, however, contains almost no enzymes when the pancreas is stimulated by secretin alone. It is the proteases and peptones in the chyme that cause the small intestine to secrete a second hormone, cholecystokinin, which is responsible for the secretion of the pancreatic digestive enzyme. The copius bicarbonate secretion by the pancreas is important in that it neutralizes acid entering the duodenum and thus provides a protective action against duodenal ulcers. **(Ref. 2,** pp. 456–458)

681. (B) The rate of gastric emptying is partially determined by the resistance to flow of the pylorus and will increase as more material is placed in the stomach. **(Ref. 2,** pp. 450–455)

682. (E) Constant vomiting can be life-threatening. The forceful expulsion of ions and fluid leads to alkalosis. A vomiting center may be located in the medulla. **(Ref. 2,** p. 211)

683. (A) Parietal cells are responsible for the secretion of HCl and intrinsic factors into the stomach. **(Ref. 2,** pp. 450–453)

684. (D) The barriers are anatomical (i.e., tight junctions in the epithelium and lack of villus membranes). **(Ref. 2,** pp. 450–455)

685. (C) The absorption of water through the intestinal membrane follows the usual laws of osmosis, therefore when the chyme is diluted, water goes from the gut lumen into the intestinal membranes. The flow is by simple diffusion. **(Ref. 2,** pp. 438–439)

686. (D) Galactose has the highest absorption rate for the carbohydrates. The absorption of one carbohydrate tends to decrease absorption for another. Transport is selective and competitive. **(Ref. 2,** pp. 433–435)

687. (E) As indicated in the question. **(Ref. 2,** pp. 442–448)

688. (E) Tactile or chemical irritation elicits reflexes that activate the enteric nervous system. Distension can elicit increased motility which in turn promotes secretion. (**Ref. 2,** pp. 442–443)

689. (B) These pangs are associated with low blood glucose levels and pain but the cause of hunger pangs is unclear, as is their contribution to the control of food intake. However, they do appear 12 to 24 hours after fasting begins and gradually weaken until they disappear after 3 or 4 days. (**Ref. 2,** pp. 453–455)

690. (B) The ninth and tenth (vagus) cranial nerves are necessary for normal swallowing. (**Ref. 2,** pp. 448–450)

691. (E) The vagus nerve supplies the striated muscle which makes up most of the upper esophagus. The middle third of this tube is mixed smooth and striated muscle while the lower third is almost entirely smooth muscle. (**Ref. 2,** pp. 448–450)

692. (A) Pepsin is secreted by the stomach, whereas trypsin, chymotrypsin, and carboxypolypeptidase are secreted by the pancreas. (**Ref. 2,** pp. 435–436)

693. (A) Protein decarboxylase and thiamine are both necessary for the decarboxylation of pyruvic acid. (**Ref. 2,** pp. 258–268)

694. (C) Pantothenic acid is a part of the co-enzyme A molecule. (**Ref. 2,** pp. 258–260, 287)

695. (B) The fat-soluble vitamin A is required for good vision. (**Ref. 2,** p. 287)

696. (E) Riboflavin (Vitamin B_2) is a crucial element in the formation of two co-enzymes that operate as hydrogen carriers within the mitochondria. (**Ref. 2,** p. 287)

697. (D) The gastric phase of digestion occurs once the food enters the stomach, and it excites the gastrin mechanism and causes local reflexes to become active. (**Ref. 2,** pp. 450–455)

698. (B) The cephalic phase of gastric secretion occurs even before food enters the stomach. Impulses from higher centers act upon the dorsal motor nuclei of the vagus which transmit excitation of the stomach. (**Ref. 2,** pp. 450–454)

699. **(D)** The mucous glands of the large intestine are regulated principally by direct tactile stimulation of the cells. (**Ref. 2,** pp. 466–470)

700. **(A)** Sympathetic stimulation of salivary glands causes vasoconstriction and results only in viscous solution to be released from the mucous portion of the glands. (**Ref. 2,** pp. 448–450)

References

1. Berne RM, Levy MN (eds.): *Physiology,* 3rd ed. Mosby Year Book, 1993.

2. Ganong WF: *Review of Medical Physiology,* 17th ed. Lange Med. Book, Appleton & Lange, 1995.